ARTS, CRAFTS AND TRADITIONAL INDUSTRIES

(Book 2)

DR. ASIM K. DASGUPTA

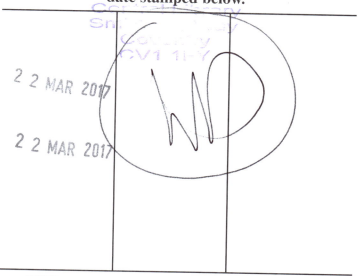

AuthorHouse™ UK Ltd.
1663 Liberty Drive
Bloomington, IN 47403 USA
www.authorhouse.co.uk
Phone: 0800.197.4150

First published by AuthorHouse January 2014
Reprinted by AuthorHouse April 2014

ISBN: 978-1-4918-8682-3(sc)
       978-1-4969-7744-1 (e)

This book is printed on acid-free paper.

Because of the dynamic nature of the Internet, any web addresses or links contained in this book may have changed since publication and may no longer be valid. The views expressed in this work are solely those of the author and do not necessarily reflect the views of the publisher, and the publisher hereby disclaims any responsibility for them.

authorHOUSE®

About the Author

DR. ASIM K. DASGUPTA is an occupational physician, now retired. He has worked as a Consultant in the United Kingdom's National Health Service and also in small and medium enterprises and in heavy industry. His work, research, and interests have taken him to many different parts of the world, and he has drawn on those travels in this book. His training, qualifications, teaching, experiences and hobbies have also played an important role in the writing of this new book on arts and crafts. He holds a medical degree from Calcutta University and a postgraduate degree (MSc) from London University. He also has a Diploma in Tropical Medicine & Hygiene from Liverpool University and a Diploma in Industrial Health from the Royal College of Physicians and Surgeons, England. He is a Member of the Faculty of Occupational Medicine (MFOM), London, and a Member of the Royal College of Physicians, London. His other book, Disasters, has already won two book awards. He lives in Hampshire, United Kingdom.

Acknowledgements

For images:
Chapter 1: image 1 by courtesy of Seema Beed and images 3 & 4 by courtesy of Stephen Ingarfill.
Chapter 7: image 4 was taken by the author with permission to use by courtesy of the Victoria & Albert Museum, London.
Chapter 14: image 2 by courtesy of Dr. Dipak Datta.
Chapter 19: images 1 & 2 by courtesy of Diego, Scotland.

My sincere thanks to those who have allowed or arranged my visits or given permission for the images that have been published in this book with a special mention to:
1. Sanjana Thawani for the quilling work,
2. Peter Crossman, Crossman crafts, Portsmouth, U.K for wooden comb making,
3. Amit and Sreyashi Kochhar for my visit to Gold Souk, Dubai,
4. Chris Imlach, Portsmouth, U.K for the buffing machine,
5. Tapan Sen, Hamen & Co., India for the sitar (Indian musical instrument),
6. Asim Dutta, Cookme, B.B.D. Pvt. Ltd., India for the spices,
7. Sayed Habib, TN Print Ltd., Portsmouth, U.K, for the printing industry,
8. Carol Bennett, Oban distillery, Oban, Scotland for the whisky industry.

For information and Library work, my thanks to the British Medical Association (BMA) Library, London; Hampshire Country Council Library, U.K; Portsmouth City Council Library, U.K and I was also dependent on the Internet search engines. However for medical literature search my special thanks to Helen Elwell of the BMA Library .

My thanks to Asoke Dasgupta for his expert view on the printing industry and Andrew Hudson for his help with the combs. Finally, I thank Dr. Rosemary Anne Williams for help in copy editing and Stephen Ingarfill for technical help.

Contents

Preface

This is my second Arts and Crafts book, in which I have described twenty more crafts. I have followed the same pattern as I used for Book 1. As I mentioned in Book 1, I have based the books on the experiences which I have gained while working, researching, travelling and visiting industries and observing arts and crafts work. From the raw materials to the finished products, I have recorded various processes and am now in a position to produce the materials in a series of books. This book is written to be easily accessible to the general public, manufacturers, apprentices, arts and crafts students and others. It will also be helpful to healthcare workers and professionals, including doctors and nurses who are interested in knowing the process and the health issues which arise from exposure to certain industries. A comment made by Kirkus Indie (U.S.A) about book 1 also applies to Book 2: 'A through guide best suited for people working in or responsible for safety and health aspects of these industries or { . . . } a starting point for those wanting to learn more.' All the photographs in this book except six (duly acknowledged) were taken by me.

Chapter 1: Bee-hive products

Bees are four-winged insects with a string. They collect nectar and pollen from flowers to produce honey and wax. A bee-hive is a structure where bees live – their home. Bees make a substance called propolis by collecting resin from bark and leaf buds, and use it to line the inside of their hives or, in the wild, their nests.

Honey can be eaten as it is, or as an ingredient in food such as cake and confectionery; it is also used in making a drink called mead. Beeswax is used to make candles, soap, polishes, and cosmetics such as cold cream, cleansing and protective creams, and depilatory creams. Propolis is used in medicinal products such as throat lozenges, tinctures, ointments, and cough syrup, or as a health product to improve immunity.

The oldest record of humans collecting honey is a prehistoric cave painting from Spain, about 15,000 years old, which shows a man climbing a cliff to access a bees' nest. Bee-keeping is recorded in antiquity.

The honeycomb is the internal structure of the bee-hive: it is a densely packed matrix of hexagonal cells made of beeswax. Honey is stored in the upper part of the comb; beneath it are the rows of pollen-storage cells, then the worker-brood cells and then the drone-brood cells. The queen cells are normally built at the lower edge of the comb. Thus in the hives there are three types of bees: the queen, which lays the eggs; the males or drones; and the workers, which feed the hive.

In the wild, bees construct natural hives made up of multiple honeycombs, usually with a single

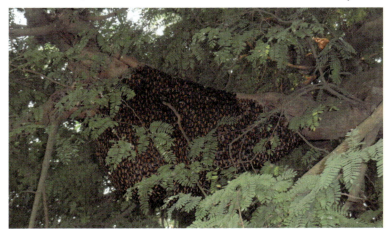

Bee-hive in the wild (India)

entrance. They are situated in tree branches, hollow trees, cliffs, caves, or rock cavities etc. Collecting wild honey can be dangerous. For example, in the mangrove swamps of the Sunderban forests of Bangladesh and West Bengal (India) honey gatherers risk attacks from the Royal Bengal Tiger. Having located a bees' nest among the tree-branches, the honey gatherers use torches made of rags or leaves and twigs to create smoke, which forces the bees to fly away.

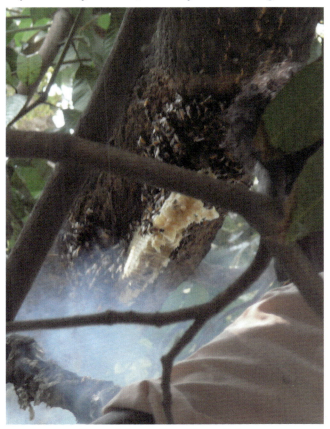

Smoking the Bee-hive

To protect themselves, the hunters cover their faces with cotton cloth, but this is inadequate. While some gatherers climb the tree and cut into the honeycomb (leaving some for future harvesting), others on the ground burst crackers and blow horns to scare away any tigers in the area. Honey flowing from the cuts in the comb is collected in bamboo baskets, which are taken away by boat.

4   In Nepal, in the forested foothills of the Himalayas, honey collectors climb up huge cliffs using bamboo ladders to access hives in crevices in the rock. As soon as a nest is located the honey hunter hoists his ladder and lights a fire. The bees, panicked by the smoke, launch a massive attack before giving up. As soon as the attack diminishes in intensity, the gatherer climbs the ladder and extracts the honey, risking a fall. With only improvised protection, gatherers' faces are often stung by the bees.

Artificial hives can be of the traditional or modern type. Traditional hives are made from mud, clay, pottery, tiles, and bee gums; modern ones of wood or plastic.
The basic components of a hive are:
a)   stand: to prevent damp and rotting wood, the hive is placed on a raised stand or on bricks;
b)   floor or bottom board: usually a flat wooden surface, with an entrance for the bees to get into the hive;
c)   brood box: the main home of the bees, where the queen bee lays her eggs;
d)   super: the uppermost box where honey is stored;
e)   queen excluder: this prevents the queen from laying eggs on top of the bees' honey store;
f)   roof: usually of wood, it protects against bad weather and prevents unwanted intrusions.

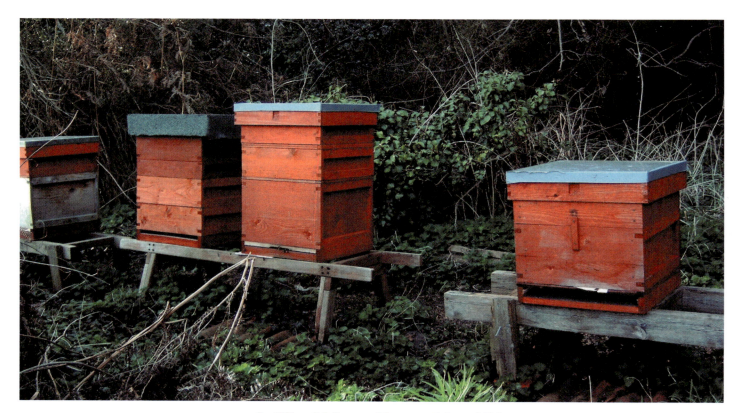

Artifical hives, Hampshire, UK

There are some variations on this basic structure. Some artificial hives have an inner cover, some an outer cover. Frames and foundations can be shorter or longer; some have handles. The commonest types of hives which are currently on the market are the Langstroth, the National, the WBC, the Commercial, the Warre, the Top Bar, the Smith, and the Dadant.
The beekeeper waits until the bees have filled the supers with honey and capped the honey-cells. Then he extracts the honey. The bees must be removed from the supers before the honey is extracted.

This is usually done by one of the following methods:

a)   using the escape board, which is placed under the super. It is essential for the super to be closely and tightly covered with a crown board or cloth;
b)   using 'fume boards' to apply chemicals such as benzaldehyde or butric anhydride; the bees recoil from the board and so leave the super;
c)   brushing away the bees, by smoking them after removing the roof and the crown board;
d)   using a mechanical blower to blow the bees out of the super.

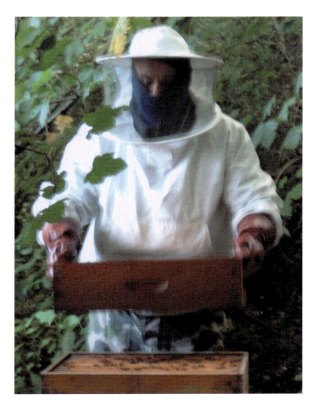

Adding a Super, while wearing protective clothing

Honey is then extracted from the frame by spinning or scraping. For spinning, a hand or electric extractor is used and a spoon is used to scrape the honey off the frame. A sharp knife is used to cut out the comb and to remove the wax capping over the surface on both sides of the frame. Finally, for a clear honey, a filter is used before bottling. The extraction process is messy: therefore a suitable room with a water supply and sink is essential. After honey, wax is the main product. It is extracted either by using a solar extractor or by using heat, water and fabric (burlap) bags. The solar extractor is an insulated container with a double-glazed lid. Wax from the hive is cut into pieces and put into the extractor. The lid then closed and the extractor is placed in the sun. When the temperature rises to 145/147°F, the wax melts and runs down the tray into the container after passing through a filter. The other method is to place small pieces of washed comb into a burlap bag and then in a cooking pot, which is heated until the comb melts and the wax escapes the bag and floats on top of the water. To achieve the highest level of purity it is necessary to repeat the process several times. Nowadays various types of stainless steel boilers are available commercially.

WHAT ARE THE HEALTH ISSUES?

1.   Bee stings can cause local or generalised hypersensitive (allergic) reactions, including bee venom allergy, hymenoptera sting reaction, beekeepers' arthopathy, nasal, eye, and respiratory allergies. The most lethal stings are those of the Africanised ('killer') bee. Bees can attack any parts of the body, but the commonest are the face and lips, causing swelling. It is possible to eliminate such reactions through desensitisation. When extracting honey and wax, beekeepers must wear head-to-foot protective clothing.
2.   Honey collectors in the wild risk injury, even death, from wild animals, or when falling from height i.e. ladders, trees, high cliffs etc.
3.   Health hazards can arise from smoke inhalation or from chemicals (benzaldehyde, butric anhydride). Cuts and burns may occur during harvesting, honey or wax processing, or during construction of artificial bee-hives. Allergic contact dermatitis from propolis, and bee-hive-dust related asthma and rhinitis, have been reported.

Chapter 2: Card and Papercraft

Card making is a kind of papercraft. Invitation cards, decorative cards, gift tags, booklets and envelopes are the common types of hand-made papercrafts, and there are many varieties ranging from card blanks to 3D greeting cards of various sizes, shapes, colours and designs. They are used to mark various festive occasions including weddings, birthdays and children's parties.

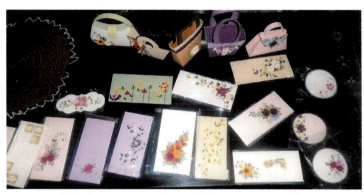

Various cards and papercrafts

Far back in history, the ancient Chinese people had a custom of sending greeting cards with goodwill messages, for example to celebrate the Chinese New Year. The ancient Egyptians used to convey greetings on papyrus scrolls. In Europe, exchanges of paper greeting cards started in the early fifteenth century. Over the last three or four decades the demand for greeting cards has been increasing worldwide. With simple techniques, paper can be transformed into beautiful greeting cards for gifts or craft objects.

The tools and some of the materials required are:

a)   paper: e.g. text, translucent, colour, hand-made, decorative, differently patterned and speciality papers,

b)   glues and adhesives,

c)   ink pads and pens, glitter and glitter pens, markers, crayons and paints,

d)   border panel strips, stitching, ribbons, beads,

e)   card toppers (made of foam, wood or metal and adhesive backing),

f)   embellishments (the commonest are ribbons, bows, stickers, beads and feathers, stuck on with glue or adhesive),

g)   outline stickers (self-adhesive stickers with personalised greetings, shapes and letters),

h)   hole punches and ink stamps of various designs,

i)   card-folding tools (bone folder, stylus, slide cutter),

j)   cutting tools (craft knives, scissors, paper trimmers, die cutters and embossing tools, shape cutters and templates),

k)   binding machine and accessories.

Which materials are used, and how, depends on the type of card. Of course design is important. Some card makers prefer to use hand-made papers. To make hand-made paper one needs: waste paper, plants, rags, decorative materials, glue and size, paints and dyes; and as equipment, a liquidizer, measuring jug, tray, sieve, mould and deckle, vat, wooden spoon, couching felts and kitchen towels, pressing boards, newspaper and non-absorbent drying material, rubber gloves and goggles.

The process is as follows:

a)   *Prepare the pulp:* make a thick pulp is made from small pieces of torn up paper, using a liquidiser and water. Pour the pulp through a sieve, and colour it using dyes or water-based paint. Then dry the pulp.

b)   *Prepare the vat and couching mound:* put the dry pulp within 3–5 litres of clean water in a rectangular tray big enough to accommodate the mould and deckle.
However, a slightly raised 'couching' mound is necessary for transferring the pulp sheet.

c)   *Make a sheet of paper:* first dampen the mesh side of the mould and place the deckle on top of it. Stir pulp with a wooden spoon, then quickly dip the mould and deckle into the vat, using a scooping movement. Remove the mould and deckle and allow them to drain.

Shake from side to side, up and down to settle the fibres. Then remove the deckle and allow the sheet of pulp to settle on the sheet of mesh.

d) *Additions to the pulp:* a variety of ingredients or decorative materials can be added to the vat or on the sheet to suit individual taste.

e) *Couch each sheet of paper:* this means transferring from the mould to a damp, thick piece of fabric which helps the paper to dry.

f) *Press, drying and size the paper:* in pressing and drying, the aim is to make sure that excess water is removed. Sizing can be done; either internally, by adding household starch or PVA (white) glue to the vat, or externally, by dissolving about one teaspoonful of gelatine or agar-agar in one litre of hot water in a shallow tray. External sizing can also be done by brushing each sheet with PVA (white) glue diluted with water.

To make a booklet card or gift tag, you will need white card, wrapping paper, glue, ruler, knife, writing paper, needle and embroidery thread. To decorate the cards the traditional technique of quilling and coiling can be used. Quilling means rolling strips of coloured paper and then squeezing them into different shapes. The art of quilling started in the fifteenth century in the Mediterranean countries.

For quilling art, quilling tools, coloured paper, coloured card, glue, hole punch, ribbon, ruler, tweezers, scissors etc. are needed and the steps are:

a) First make the individual quills. This is done by cutting strips of coloured paper and then rolling them up individually, starting from one end, using a quilling tool.

b) Once the roll is complete, let it uncoil slightly, then glue the end and hold it.

c) A coiled and glued strip can be shaped into many traditional forms: circle, triangle, pear shape, eye, scroll and so on.

d) Finally, make a pattern by arranging the quills on a piece of folded card in a good background colour.

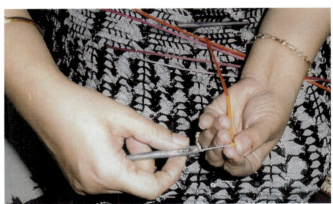

Quilling work

Punch a hole in the card with a hole punch and thread a ribbon through the hole to make a miniature card or gift tag. Some special types of cards are made by using advanced techniques such as a) embossing (raising areas within the paper, card or foil on cards), b) parchment craft (embossing and piercing vellum paper to give the appearance of lace), c) aperture cards (which have a widow or aperture in the middle), d) Shaker cards (gluing together two pieces of transparent thin card or vellum), e) Computer-generated cards have become popular recently

WHAT ARE THE HEALTH ISSUES?

Tool-related finger injuries have been reported, as have wet-hand-related electrical shock injuries. Material-related skin and respiratory disorders (irritant and allergic phenomena) can occur. Paper dust may cause increased episodes in sufferers from asthma, bronchitis, emphysema or chronic obstructive airways diseases. The paper and pulp industries are known to be associated with increased risk of certain cancers (lung, stomach, lymphomas), obstructive lung disease and bronchitis, but here risk is less than in the paper and pulp industries because there is less exposure. Self-protection is important (gloves, apron, and respirator) and a well-ventilated room is essential, especially when using paints, dyes and plant fibres. Cramp, musculoskeletal disorders and twisting injuries can occur. The dexterous hand movements necessary for quilling may result in upper limb disorders.

Chapter 3: Clock and watch making

Clocks and watches are for 'timekeeping'. The ancient world relied on sun, moon and shadows for time and calendar calculation. This led to various types of sun-god worship, and to the use of sundials.

The mechanical clock was first invented about the mid-thirteenth century, and since then over the centuries the processes for manufacturing clocks and watches have made tremendous progress. Switzerland is famous for watch and clock manufacturing.

Any mechanical clock, whether big or small, and all wrist watches work on the same principle, in accordance with the laws of physics. To operate, they need a source of power, and hands to indicate or measure the time.

The power source is mainly one of three kinds: a falling weight, a coiled spring, or electricity. Grandfather clocks, tower clocks, church clocks and those in other public buildings usually use falling weight or weight-driven devices for power.

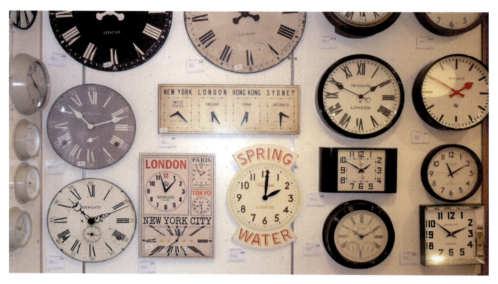

Clocks on a wall

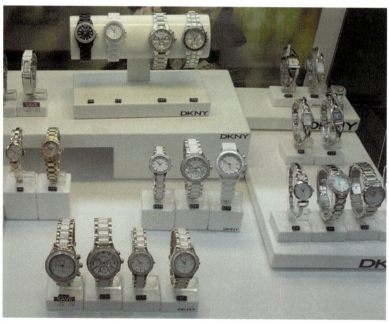

Watches on display

Small clocks and most watches are powered by a coiled spring which needs winding; the disadvantage is that it gradually loses its power as the spring uncoils. To avoid spring problems, the clocks incorporate an extra device such as a fusee, escapement, regulator and so on. A fusee is a spirally grooved pulley that is used to equalise the pull of the mainspring. The mainspring is usually regulated by a balance wheel fitted with a hairspring.

An escapement is a part of the clock that links the oscillator (pendulum or a balance) to the power source and thus controls the rate. The regulator is a device which ensures a steady regular movement; the commonest types are the pendulum and the balance wheel. The balance wheel and the escape wheels are some of the moving parts of the watch that need a bearing in order to turn. The hardest bearings are jewelled bearings.

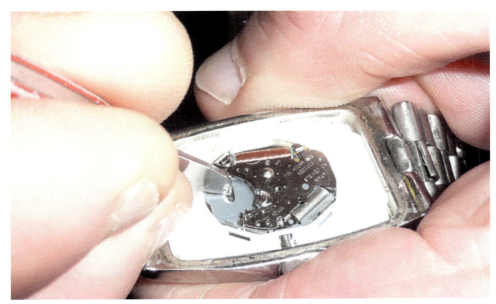

Some watches also use vibrations from a tuning fork, or from certain crystals or atoms. Nowadays most watches are powered by a battery, and clocks are mostly electric, including large public clocks. These clocks are not only powered by electricity but also regulated by it. Most modern watches consist of hour and minute hands as well as second hands. Some also show the date and day, many are automatic.

Electronic watch components

It is important that clocks and watches should maintain accurate timing. For precision time keeping the *chronometer* is used; it incorporates a fusee mechanism. *Quartz crystal clocks* are among the most accurate timepieces; the crystals have electrical properties making them suitable for regulating the mechanism of a clock. The thinner the crystal, the faster it vibrates. A better type for accurate timekeeping is the *atomic clock*, in which one of the substances used is caesium whose atoms vibrate very rapidly and regularly.

Nowadays watches are also available with shock resistance, water resistance, anti-magnetic properties, alarms and luminous numerals. Luminous watches are popular among military personnel and underwater divers. In the last century, in making luminous watches, the luminous paint used by women was highly radioactive and therefore carcinogenic. Since 1960, non-radioactive materials such as photoluminescent materials have been used. They are zinc sulphide, strontium aluminates and tritium. Nowadays most watch manufacturers use tritium tube technology, i.e. tiny glass tubes containing gaseous tritium. Luxury watches are also becoming popular. However the demand for high precision, high quality devices is increasing.

To make a watch there are three basic components:

a) An inside component that can measure time accurately to the nearest second using oscillations, whose quantity is defined in hertz. The number of parts varies from 200 to 400. They include levers, base plates, bridges, balance wheels, hairsprings, shock absorbers, nuts and rivets.

b) Dial: to make a dial, one should start with the initial design, giving importance to the colour of the dial, the lettering and the variations of positioning. Once the style is selected, it must be translated into technical drawings. The next stage is manufacturing. Some manufactures use a laser and sapphire glass to make the dial. The object is to cut the sapphire glass stone to the correct size, height and specification. The resulting disc must have a perfectly transparent surface. This is achieved by polishing. Then comes enamelling and baking in an oven at a temperature of about 800°C. When it is taken out of the oven, the manufactured dial is complete.

c) Cases and watch bands/straps: many clock cases are made of wood. Precious and non-precious metals are generally used for watch cases. Watch straps, watch bands and watch

10 bracelets can be made of metal or of non-metallic materials. These include leather, textile, silicones, rubber and plastic.

d)   The final process is the assembling of all these three.

Some parts require extremely precise manufacturing. Hence, in the clock and watch industry, high percentages of women are employed because they have smaller hands, suitable for precise work.

Some of the common tools used in clock and watch making are hammers, pliers, files, vice, screwdrivers, tweezers, bushes, cutting tools, winding tools, measuring tools, magnetic pick up tools, measuring tools, bench and abrasive, adhesive, oils and polishing tools.

Computerised machine technology today has replaced the traditional manually operated equipment. This technology includes computer-aided design software (CAD) and computer numerical control (CNC) machines. Some are used to grind sapphire glasses, some produce complex engraving and others are used in base plate manufacturing. Lesser machines are used for smaller molten-metal tasks.

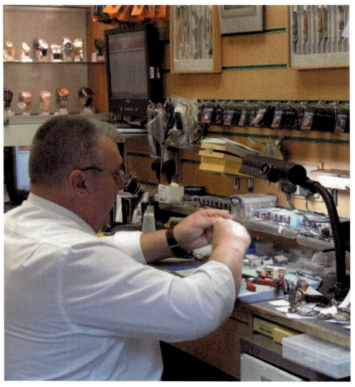

Watchmaker

Automation has replaced manpower – the long hours of work as well as the hand skills of watch makers. The single watchmaker sitting at an old-fashioned bench and often working on the watch from start to finish is now rare. High-tech assembly lines have replaced the traditional conveyor belt shuttling carriages containing watch parts around the shop floor.

Some operations are performed by robots: for example, oiling and measuring. Automation is used to relieve human beings of repetitive tasks, but some complex assembly still relies on manual skills.

Some of the most famous watch manufacturers, like Omega and Rolex, use mostly computerised technology and are based in Switzerland.

WHAT ARE THE HEALTH ISSUES?

Tool- or equipment-related injuries, including mainspring-related tension injuries, can occur. Burns, eyestrain and noise-related health issues and fire hazards exist. Posture-related muscular disorders and workstation-related ergonomic factors may cause problems amongst clock and watch makers. Muscle fatigue and other upper limb disorders, including repetitive strain injuries as a result of operations requiring manual dexterity or dexterity with the fingers, can occur. Cleaning and lubricating materials, specifically solvents, oil and grease, are associated with skin and respiratory disorders. Handling nickel, mercury, dyestuffs and gold plate (cyanide) is no doubt toxic to watch makers. Quartz- and metal-related dust hazards include silicosis and other respiratory disorders. Since the 1960s or early 1970s, no more radium materials have been used for self-luminous parts of watches and clocks, which means that cancers related to radium dial painting, and 'radiation jaw', are now mostly history.

Chapter 4: Comb making

A comb is a kind of toothed tool or device, used mainly in hair care, for delousing, decorating, cleaning, and tidying the hair. A nit comb is a specialised type of comb which is used to remove parasites such as lice, fleas, mites, and fungal growths from hair. In industry, combs are used to separate cotton fibres from seeds and debris; they also used to distribute colour in paper marbling (making marbled patterns on paper) and for making music notes in the music industry. Sometimes combs are used for forensic purposes, such as to collect hair in police investigations etc.

Comb making is an ancient craft whose history goes back to the Stone Age. The first hair-comb, made of animal bone with four teeth, radio-carbon dated to 8000 BC, was excavated on the bank of the River Euphrates in Syria. Combs are universal and found all over the world, used by every culture and civilisation. Combs have thin or fine teeth that are spaced very close together. There may or may not be a handle (narrow tail on one end). Utility-wise, hair combs can be classified into two categories: a) utilitarian and b) decorative or ornamental. They may be made from various types of materials such as wood, bone and antler, horn, ivory, metal, plastic, tortoise shell, amber, coral, jade, pearls, spun glass, and so on. Animal bone, horn, ivory, or tortoise shell, which were once quite popular, are now rarely used because of animal conservation issues. Nowadays the main materials are plastic, wood, or metal. Types of tools, equipment, and processes depend on the types of materials that are used.

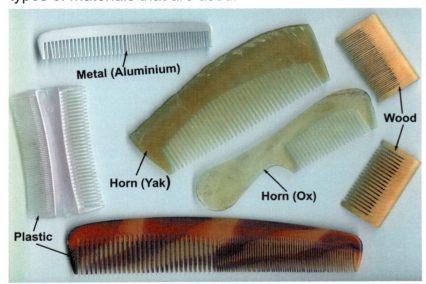

Metal (Aluminium)

Horn (Yak)

Horn (Ox)

Wood

Plastic

Combs made of horn, wood, metal and plastic

For making plastic combs, injection moulding techniques are used and the plastic materials are cellulose nitrate, cellulose acetate, nylon, polypropylene, butyrate, and polystyrene (high impact). The equipment which is used consists of:
a) injection moulding machine,
b) scrap grinder for recycled plastics (plastic granules),
c) clamping units,
d) buffing, polishing, and stamping machine,
e) mould releasing agent, lubricant, and packaging material.

The process is as follows:
The cellulose nitrate sheet or the polypropylene granules are fed into the hopper of an injection-moulding system. The mould is held between the two clamping units. The materials injected into the mould are elasticized under high pressure, resulting in a moulded comb. After cooling, the mould is opened and the comb ejected; this is followed by buffing, polishing, stamping, and finally packaging.

For wooden combs, hard woods are used and the choice of woods depends on whatever suitable local woods are available. Thus, in tropical and sub-tropical countries tropical hardwoods such as fruitwoods are used. In Britain and other European countries the main types of wood are boxwood *(Buxus sempervirens)*, holly *(Ilex aquifolians)*, hornbeam *(Carpinus betulus)*, pear *(Pyrus communis)*, crab apple, and beech.

12 To make a wooden comb the main tools used are:

1) rasp (for shaping the block gauge),
2) marking gauge (for setting the tooth depth),
3) saws (single and double bladed, to cut teeth),
4) files (triangular and wedge shaped, to shape the teeth or form),
5) sanding agent (*equisetum hyemale* – the scouring rush – sand, sandpaper, or heather),
6) bee's wax, for finishing,
7) knives,
8) work bench (as a steady base).

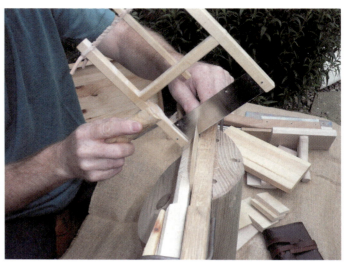

Cutting teeth –wooden comb

The process involves:

Step one: *blocking out*, i.e. making a square block mark with centre lines on the hardwood.

Step two: *shaping block*, i.e. shaping up the square block using rasps.

Step three: *marking block*, i.e. marking tooth depth using a the marking gauge.

Step four: *cutting teeth*, using a saw or 'stadda' (twin-bladed saw).

Step five: *grailing*, i.e. filing the teeth to a point.

Step six: *finishing*, i.e. sanding and waxing.

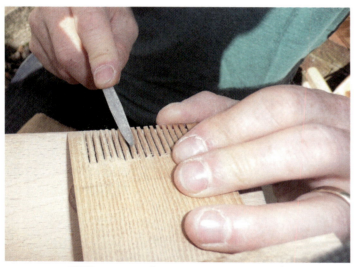

Filing teeth - wooden comb

For making metal combs, metals like steel, aluminium, brass, bronze, copper, gold, and silver are used. To shape the metal into a comb, the techniques of casting, moulding, beating, cutting, trimming, grinding and polishing, etc. are used; but with the introduction of mechanisation, the individual manual techniques and skills of comb making have disappeared or are disappearing. In India, the filigree technique is used to produce combs from very fine wire, usually gold, silver, or brass.

WHAT ARE THE HEALTH ISSUES?

The health issues largely depend on the type of comb that one is making. For example, during the plastic-comb-making process burns, injuries, and noise-related physical hazards, as well as skin disorders (contact dermatitis) and respiratory disorders (allergic and irritant), can occur. Cuts and injuries also occur from handheld tools during wood and metal comb making. Hand injuries, especially to the non-dominant hand, are more common amongst wood-comb makers. Noise hazards are more significant during sheet metal shaping. Metal comb makers are at risk from respiratory, musculo-skeletal, and skin disorders, whereas wood-comb makers are more likely to suffer from wood-dust-related skin disorders (dermatitis) or respiratory disorders (allergic and irritant). Cancer has not been reported amongst comb makers, but there are concerns about wood dust and cancers related to plastic materials (polypropylene and acetate).

Chapter 5: Coral and seashell products

Sea products like coral and shells are one of the world's most popular craft-making industries. The industry is so popular that there may be some scarcity or extinction issues.

There are many types of sea shells, including gastropods (snails, conches, cowries, whelks, periwinkles), bivalves (pelecypods, clams, mussels, oysters, scallops, cockles), cephalopods (squids, octopuses, chambered nautilus), scaphopods (tusk shells, captacula), and molluscs like chitons and amphineura which are found on beaches.

These are the empty shells from many dead marine animals whose soft bodies rot away, after which the shells are often washed ashore. Shells are found in various shapes and sizes. Coral and coral reefs are found in shallow tropical waters.

Corals can be hard or soft. Hard corals are limestone skeletons which make various shapes on the reef and named accordingly as Table, Brain, Mushroom and Black corals. Soft corals are those that do not have a hard skeleton; they usually grow in various colours such as red, yellow, pink and purple. The types are named according to their appearance: for example, Fan corals, Whip corals, Fire corals and Feeding corals.

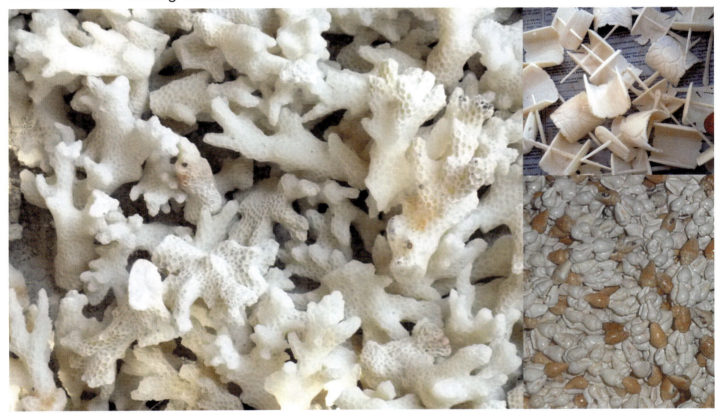

Coral and seashell products including cowrie

History tells us that since the beginning of the Stone Age, humans have collected shells and used them as tools, weapons, vessels, musical instruments, jewellery, currency and decorative uses. A conch-shell trumpet was the first musical instrument, made by making a hole in the side of the shell. Cowrie has been used as a currency in various parts of the world, thanks to its lightness, durability, ease of transport and convenience for trade. In ancient Egypt, Rome, Africa, the Mediterranean area and Asia, cowrie was used in religious festivals, in folk customs, and for protection, as it symbolised fertility, birth and womanhood.

14 Conus shell was used as forehead jewellery in Central Africa and was also used as bracelets by the ancient Egyptians. Sophisticated craft-making techniques using shells and coral started during the Renaissance, and without a doubt it has become a most popular arts and crafts industry in modern days.

To make crafts with coral, several types of artistic techniques are used. Coral beads, chips, jewellery (bracelets, necklaces, earrings and anklets), key chains, napkin rings and decorative objects for the home are some of the common artefacts made by coral craft.

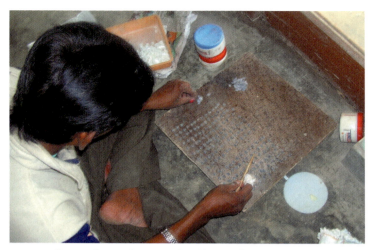

Coral and seashell craft working

Similarly, the artefacts made from shells include jewellery, furniture, curtains, ornaments, candles, buttons, decorative hats, clothing, mirrors, clocks, home and building decorations including shell mosaics, grottos, cards and albums.

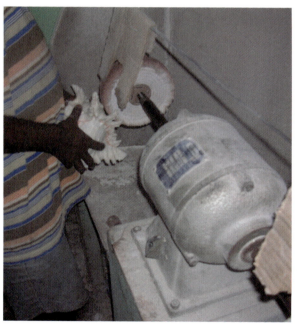

Polishing the conch shell

To make such artefacts, apart from coral and sea shells, other items of equipment and materials are necessary. They are: craft knife, drill, grinder, files, hammer, hole punch, saw, scalpel, scissors, screwdriver, screw, nails, bolts, brackets, hooks, hinges, tweezers, wire cutters, thread, epoxy resins, glue, adhesive, tapes, paint and brushes, and so on.

These items are used for
1) drilling (ordinary drill for large shells, mini drills for small shells),
2) grinding (pointed grinder for grinding the inside of shells such as scallops; straight-edge grinder to smooth the rough edge of the shell),
3) sawing (hacksaw for flat scallops),
4) sanding, with a coarse- and a fine-grade sanding disc,
5) polishing by various mop heads, made of felt, wool or cotton,
6) varnishing,
7) painting so that beautiful seashell and coral crafts or objects are produced.

WHAT ARE THE HEALTH ISSUES?

There may be tool- or machine-related issues including noise, and eye and hand injuries. Similarly cuts and abrasions can be caused by dead coral, and infection is the main concern. Precautions are to be taken when handling poisonous conch shells; the sting can cause mainly local reaction, but nausea, faintness, palpitations or breathing difficulties can occur. Coral dermatitis, dust-related allergies and respiratory disorders are known health issues. Risks of respiratory tract disorders are associated with drilling, grinding, sawing and sanding the coral and sea shells; on the other hand, skin-related disorders are associated with varnishing and painting of those products. Epoxy-resin-related skin and dust disorders, hot glue burns and fire-related hazards can occur.

Trees consist of bark and wood. Bark is used in cork-making industries as the cork is the prime substance of the bark tissue which is harvested from the evergreen oak tree (*Quercus suber*). So, the components of the bark tissue are outer bark, cork and the inner bark. Because of its buoyancy, elasticity, and fire resisting properties, cork has many uses. It is used in wine or other bottle stoppers, flooring materials (linoleum), roofing panels, bulletin boards, dart boards, fishing rods, floats, buoys, musical instruments, shoes and other footwear, baseballs, golf and cricket balls, cork hats and heat shields, safety helmet liners, and so on.
The earliest findings of cork products are cork bottle stoppers in ancient Egyptian tombs.

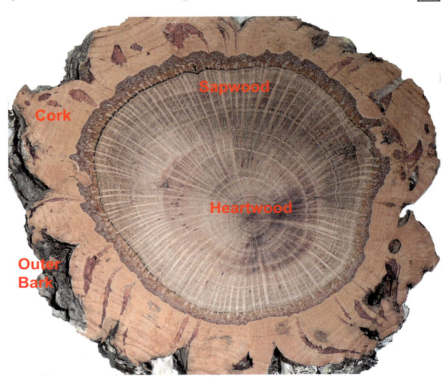

Cross section of the oak trunk

The ancient Greeks also used cork as bottle stoppers, saddle liners, and fishing-net floats; the ancient Romans used it for fishermen's life jackets.

Over the years the roofs and floors of Mediterranean houses have been built with cork to protect from severe cold and heat. From the 17th-18th century onwards the cultivation of cork trees increased because of high demand for cork stoppers.

Spain, Portugal, Algeria, France, Italy, and Tunisia are the main cork-producing countries; 45-50% of the world's cork is harvested by Portugal.

The cork is usually cut from the trees and cork extraction is a specialised job: the cork is usually separated from the tree without damaging the tree permanently.

1. Harvesting:
Harvesting time is usually May to late August. The first cork harvesting is done when the tree reaches about 25–30 years of age and the trunk circumference is 60 cm (24 inches). Subsequent cork extractions are done every 9–12 years. The life span of a cork-oak tree is at least 159 years.

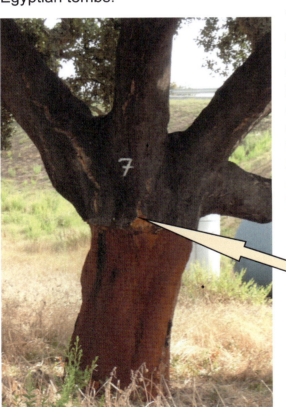

Cork trees after cork extraction

Inset of cork cutting point showing bark tissue

16   The worker or extractor uses a very sharp axe or hatchet, and they make two types of cut: one horizontal and one vertical. The art of extraction is to detach the cork without damaging the tree. Using the wedge-shaped handle of the hatchet, the harvester strips each panel of cork from the tree. The cork is stacked and then loaded on to a truck and dispatched to a processor.

2. Production process:

In the factory yard, the cork planks are stacked outdoors for between a few weeks and six months as a part of the curing processing; the air, sun, and rain encourage chemical changes that improve the quality of the cork. After this curing process the planks are flattened out and are boiled to remove dirt and other water-soluble components (tannin).

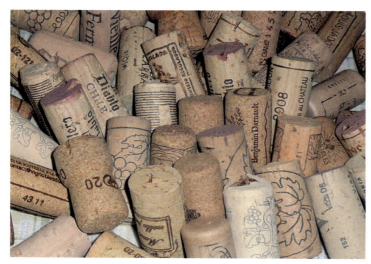

Cork wine stoppers

Further process involves treating the cork planks with fungicide: this is done by lowering them into large copper vats filled with boiling water containing fungicide for one hour, totally submerged. The planks are then removed from the vat and the poor-quality outer layer of cork is scraped off with a knife. The planks are then stacked in a dark cellar for few more weeks and allowed to dry and cure under controlled humidity. Inside the factory, they are cut into strips by circular saws and trimmed to a uniform, rectangular shape. They are then sorted on the basis of quality. The best qualities are used to make wine-bottle stoppers etc. and the poor quality-material will be ground and used for making agglomerated cork.

Corks are punched from the cork strips by either hand punching or machine punching. Punching is done with a sharp, cylindrical knife. The knife determines the cork's width; the height determines its length. Unused cork scraps and dust are collected for processing into other cork products such as insulation and construction materials. The corks are washed, bleached, and sterilized in large vats. Chemical bathing is used to condition the corks: either a) a chlorinated lime bath followed by a neutralising bath of oxalic acid, or b) a hypochlorite bath neutralised by sodium oxalate, or c) a peroxide bath neutralised with citric acid. The corks are then dried in the centrifuge dyer, graded, and marked. The corks are sorted manually, whereby eyesight is important. The marking is done using ink or a hot metal stamp. Some corks are also coated with paraffin or silicone. Then they are packed in airtight bags in batches. To keep the corks more sterile, air is usually removed from the bags and replaced with sulphur dioxide (SO_2).

WHAT ARE THE HEALTH ISSUES?

Respiratory disorders are the main health issues. Cork-related asthma (cork-workers' asthma), bronchitis and suberosis are such respiratory disorders. Suberosis is a type of hypersensitive pneumonitis or asthma caused by exposure to cork proteins and moulds such as *Aspergillus fumigatus* and *Penicillium frequentans*. Harvesting- and machinery-related physical injuries can occur. Appropriate precautions must be taken against skin disorders (dermatitis), dangers to eyesight, noise hazards and chemical burns that one might find in cork industries.

Chapter 7: Doll making

A doll is a model of a human figure, and to produce it throughout the ages a wide range of materials has been used: bone, clay, terracotta, china, corn husks, cloth, paper, papier-mâché, leather, plastic, polymers, vinyl, porcelain, rubber, resin, wax, wood, stone, plaster, cement, polyester and so on. Children use dolls as toys.

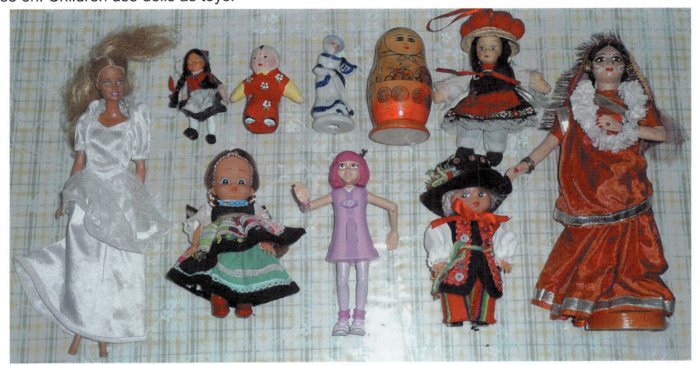

Fashion doll (Barbie) and dolls made of porcelain, wood, fabric, plastic and clay.

The processes involve modelling, firing, mould making, casting, carving and finishing. Of course the process largely depends on the types of material used. These also determine what tools and doll-making accessories will be required.

Looking back through history, we find that dolls have traditionally been used in magic, spiritual or religious rituals. Such traditional dolls are found in Africa, Asia, America and Europe and are usually made of clay, wood, straw or corn husks. Dolls are also documented in ancient civilisations, including Egypt in 2000 BC, Japan in 8000–200 BC, Rome in 300 BC and Greece in 100 AD. Modern doll manufacturing started in Germany in the fifteenth century. With industrialisation mass production of dolls with raw materials such as porcelain, and the use of leather, cloths, papier mâché and other composite materials, began. From the twentieth century onwards, with the advance of plastics, polymers and synthetic resins, dolls became extremely popular. Children love to play with dolls, especially dolls with movable limbs, removable clothing or combable hair. Fashion dolls, action figures, art dolls and entertainment dolls are the types of dolls which are manufactured by the various countries of the world. With the introduction of computers and the advance of the internet, more life-like or realistic dolls are available nowadays.

Fashion dolls include Bisque, Barbie, Bratz and Blythe.

Entertainment dolls are mainly for children's circus shows, puppet shows, or for certain craft activities. One of the most famous classes of puppet dolls is Rajasthani string puppets. These dolls have painted wooden heads and are draped with dresses made from old fabrics. The hands are made by stuffing rags or cotton into the sleeves of the dress. The most important thing is to produce an expression; this is usually done by painting large expressive eyes with arched eyebrows and, for a male, a curling moustache; for the woman, a nose ring.

A doll's house is a toy home, usually made in a miniature form. It is usually a plywood or fibre-wood cabinet with several rooms, furnished with miniature furniture and accessories that accommodate dolls of the correct size. Although it existed in some form in the ancient world, the origins of the modern doll's house are in Europe, dating back to the sixteenth or seventeenth century.

Dolls can be articulated or non-articulated. Non-articulated dolls are usually all-in-one dolls and are simple to make. Whatever the type of doll, a basic knowledge of anatomy, design, sculpturing, moulding etc. is necessary to produce good dolls. To construct a doll, one has to select the materials first, and design body parts like the head, face, torso, arms and legs. So doll construction involves:

Head: to make the head one first has to decide the head type. Does it need curving or sculpturing or casting or moulding? Is it to be a shoulder head or a swivel head or a socket head or a flange neck head? The next step is to decide the materials, which could be wood, paper pulp, paper, wax, stoneware or marble, bisque, cloth or rags, felt, porcelain, metal, celluloid, vinyl or various other types of plastics which are available nowadays.

Body: to make female bodies, it is important to shape the body so that it shows the breasts, waist, hips and bottom. When the doll's body is designed, besides the shape other features are to be considered, such as type of head, its jointing and mobility. Materials used to make bodies are usually the same as for the head, but different types of materials could be used. For example, the body is made of stuffed cloth but the head is made of wax. Using the moulding technique, the composition of the body is usually hollow and the cast is done in two halves (front and back) which are then joined together.

Limbs: generally there are two types of limbs to be considered: either complete or divided. The complete limb is from the shoulders to the fingers, or from hips to toes. The divided limb is usually in three components: for the arm it is divided into upper, lower and hand; for the leg it is divided into upper, lower and foot. Jointing is necessary to assemble the different parts of limbs, but for a complete limb no jointing is necessary. A bent limb is usually a complete limb and is made of vinyl or other plastic materials. The vinyls are cast in moulds and casts are done as one unit, instead of in two halves like bodies.

Face and hair: to design dolls' heads the shape of the face, facial features and hair are all important. Faces can be round, long, square or heart shaped; this largely depends on the imagination of the doll maker. Besides shape, the head needs to have two eyes, two ears, a nose and a mouth, created on bone structures including the forehead, brows, checks, chin and jaws. Eyes can be painted, glass, or be sleeping eyes with provision for movement. The mouth is usually created bearing in mind whether it is to be open, smiling, or showing teeth or tongue. To produce such effects, a moulding technique is sometimes used. The next thing is to create a nose, which largely depends on the material used; an attractive nose changes the overall look of the doll. The ears are usually made either as part of the back of the head or as a part of a moulded head that has been cast along with the face. Using real hair is the most common way to produce attractive dolls, but not all dolls are designed to have hair. Many heads are moulded to show hair; sometimes curls are

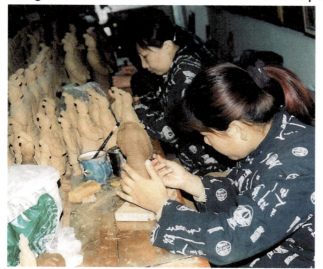

Clay doll working

painted on the head. Real hair can be either human or animal. Other materials are nylon or mohair. The hair is usually inserted through small holes into the head and then knotted. Nylon or mohair can be made as wigs. However nylon is more popular as hair for modern mass-produced dolls. Although dolls can be made from many different materials, the art of doll making is becoming more popular with the use of plastic-based vinyl, resin or polymers.

Polymer dolls are usually made from polymer clay. After determining the general size and shape of the polymer doll, a wire (steel)

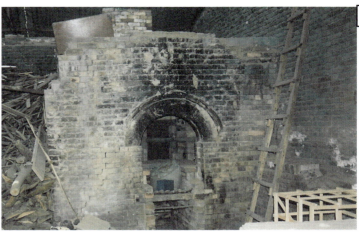

Clay doll firing kiln

skeleton or armature must be made. When making the limbs, torso and head, cut off any excess wire with wire cutters, and add aluminium foil to fill up some of the bulk of the body shape. Wrap aluminium foil around the top of the torso wire for the head and add it for the body and limbs. Coat the armature with polyvinyl glue. Once it is dried, cover it with polymer clay. Then gradually build up the head, neck, body and limbs. To make the appropriate shape, scoop out areas that need depth and add portions of clay where bulk is needed. Sculpt the neck, face and other parts of the body and limbs by pushing and pulling the clay, and create the facial features, fingers and toes. Clay or sculpture tools may be needed. Place and bake the doll in the oven, keeping in mind the appropriate time and temperature. When the baking is finished, take the doll out of the oven and leave it to cool. Remove the undesirable surface texture by sanding the doll lightly. Paint or colour the doll; acrylic paints are used for this. To add hair and clothing, hair materials, fabrics, sewing needles, knitting needles and scissors are needed.

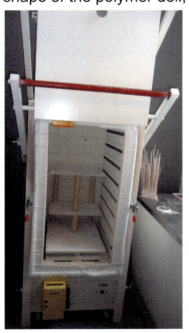

Oven for firing dolls

WHAT ARE THE HEALTH ISSUES?

Respiratory, eye and skin hazards may arise in the form of occupational asthma, rhinitis, conjunctivitis and contact dermatitis; it depends on what types of materials are handled. The most popular materials are plastic-based vinyl, resin or polymers. Vinyl chloride has a toxic effect on the nervous system (headache, light-headedness, dizziness), on vascular and skeletal systems (Raynaud's phenomenon, scleroderma-like skin lesions, acro-osteolysis), and on the hepatic system (hepatitis, cirrhosis) and the respiratory system (asthma, pneumonitis, pulmonary fibrosis). There is also a risk of liver, brain or blood cancer. Resins can cause asthma, rhinitis and dermatitis. Resin-related risk of cancer affects the lung and pancreas. Polymer fume fever results from inhalation of polymer products and can manifest both immediate symptoms (dry throat, rhinitis, chest tightness and conjunctivitis) and late symptoms (fever, chills and myalgias). Acrylic-paint-related hazards include dermatitis, asthma and peripheral neuropathy. Work-related upper limb disorders as a result of pushing and pulling, as well as tools-related injuries, are not uncommon. Burn-related injuries are usually associated with firing or baking the dolls.

Chapter 8: Gemstones

Gemstones are naturally occurring minerals that are available in the form of precious and semi-precious stones. There are many types of gemstones; they are identified by their chemical composition and are classified on the basis of colour, translucency, hardness and crystal structure.

Precious stones are natural stones which are characterised by their colour, transparency, brilliancy, durability (whether they are hard enough to be difficult to break or scratch) and rarity. They are:

Diamond – carbon, cubic structure with hardness of 10. Most diamonds are colourless, but yellow, brown, red, pink, grey, black, blue and green diamonds are also found.

Emerald – beryllium aluminium silicate, hexagonal structure with hardness of 7.5. The colour of emerald is green and it belongs to the beryl group.

Ruby – aluminium oxide, trigonal structure with hardness of 9. Red is the usual colour, but pinkish, purplish or brownish red are also available.

Sapphire – aluminium oxide, trigonal structure with hardness of 9. The most valuable colour is deep blue, but variations on this blue colour are also available.

Topaz – aluminium fluorohydroxysilicate, orthorhombic structure with hardness of 8. Colours are golden yellow, pink, blue and green.

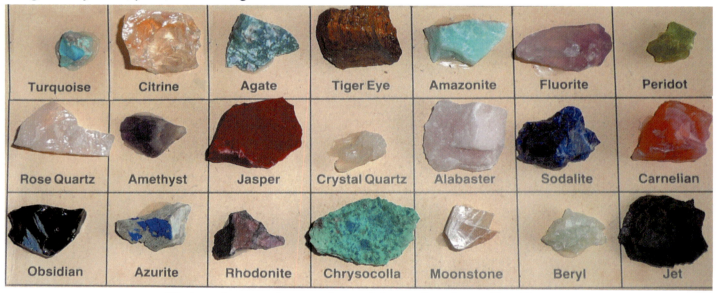

Natural gemstones (rough)- author's collection

Semi-precious stones are also naturally occurring stones but they have some deficiencies which prevent them being as good as precious stones. Some of the common stones are:

Agate – silicon dioxide, trigonal structure of chalcedony quartz with hardness of 7, found in a variety of colours and textures.

Amethyst – silicon dioxide, trigonal structure, one of the quartz group with hardness of 7; the colour varies from pale lilac to deep reddish purple.

Citrine – silicon dioxide, trigonal structure with hardness of 7; the colour is yellow to gold. Belongs to the quartz group.

Turquoise – hydrated copper aluminium phosphate, a triclinic structure with hardness of 6. The colour varies from sky blue to green.

Jasper – silicon dioxide, trigonal structure with hardness of 7. Fine-grained chalcedony with shades of brown, red, yellow, green and greyish blue.

Peridot – magnesium iron silicate, orthorhombic structure with hardness of 6.5; the colour is olive or bottle green.

Moonstone – potassium aluminium silicate, monoclinic structure with hardness of 6. The colour is milky white, or with a blue shine like the moon.

The main gem producing countries are Afghanistan, Australia, Brazil, Botswana, China, Colombia, Czech Republic, East Africa, Egypt, Germany, Italy, India, Mexico, Myanmar, Madagascar, Pakistan, Russia, South Africa, Sri Lanka, Thailand, Zambia, Zaire and USA.

Gemstones were first used by Stone Age men to make tools (obsidian axes) and since then human civilisation has always attached importance to using gemstones to make jewellery, to make ornamental or decorative clothing, in medicine, and for good luck and protection. In modern days they are used in industries, especially quartz watches, industrial tools, machines with electrical conductors, electronics and credit cards.

Gemstone making involves several processes. Once the gemstone is mined, it undergoes washing and drying processes. Once it is dried, the next steps are slicing and grinding. Knowing the hardness of the gemstones is important during slicing or grinding. Sometimes resin is used to prevent cracking. Finishing is done by sanding and polishing.

The basic principles or techniques behind gem making are as follows:

1)   *Hardness*: when working with gemstones it is important to know their durability, resistance to scratching, and ability to take and retain the polish. For that each gemstone is graded for hardness using the Mohs scale (01 – Talc, 02 – Gypsum, 03 – Calcite, 04 – Fluorspar, 05 – Apatite, 06 – Orthoclase, 07 – Quartz, 08 – Topaz, 09 – Corundum, and 10 – Diamond). This is essential if gemstones are to be cut and set in jewellery.

2)   *Shapes and cuts*: the cutting and shaping of semi-precious and precious stones is called lapidary work. Shapes and cuts are done in two ways:
a) when a cut is simple it is called cabochon;
b) when a stone surface is cut into a number of flat faces this is called faceting and it is done with a faceting machine. Grinding wheels and polishing agents are used to grind, shape and polish the stones and the faceting machine is used to hold the stone on a flat surface for cutting and polishing the flat facets.

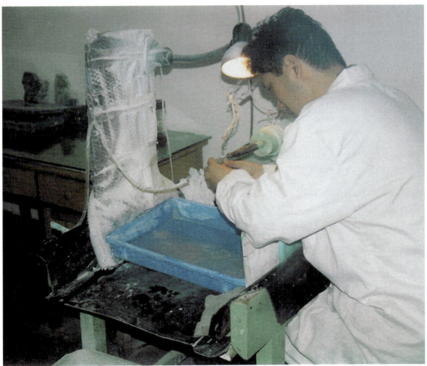

Lapidary work

3) *Colour and lustre*: colour is the most important characteristic of gemstones. Some gemstones are colourless; some retain their colours always, some most of the time, and some only in the right conditions. The colour of a gemstone depends on the way it absorbs the light. When light passes through a gem, some colours are absorbed but some are not: they are reflected back and give the gem its colour or lustre. Lustre is determined by the way the light is reflected from the, surface which is in turn related to the degree of surface polish.

4) *Polishing, carving, engraving and settings*: polishing means giving a shine to the stone; it is done by rubbing it with another stone, or with powder or grit. Carving means cutting gemstones from larger pieces of material, and it is usually done using a chisel or turning machine. Engraving means making holes, lines or other decorations on the surface of the gemstones. It is usually done using a driller, graver etc. Setting means to hold, attach or secure a gemstone with metal, plastic, or other less conventional materials. There are various types of settings and tools, and processes vary according to the setting style.

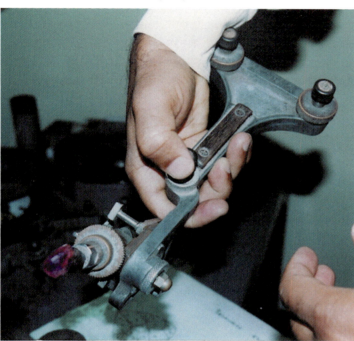

Finished gemstone (Ruby)

5) *Waxing, oiling and gemstone treatment*: the terms waxing/oiling are applied when the natural fissures of gemstones are filled with wax or oil. When a gemstone is fractured, the fracture filling is done with lead glass. To improve the colour or clarity of the gemstones, they undergo a heating process, or oil and chemical treatment. Cider oil, synthetic oil, and polymers are some of the oils or chemicals which are used.

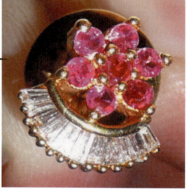

Finished rubies in 'settings'

WHAT ARE THE HEALTH ISSUES?

Besides noise and vibration, upper-limb, neck- and back-related ergonomic hazards are the main concern during gemstone mining. Eyestrain and physical injuries amongst child labourers in gem polishing have been reported. Eyestrain includes symptoms like itching, burning or irritated eyes, tired or heavy eyes, blurring or double vision, and headache due to improper lighting or illumination. Drillers, grinders, polishers and buffers are exposed to gemstone dust. High prevalence of respiratory disorders, including silicosis, has been reported. Risks of cobalt-related asthma and pulmonary fibrosis are a threat to gem polishers in the diamond industry who use cobalt-faced polishing disks. The use of glues, epoxy resin and plastic materials can lead to hand dermatitis and other toxic hazards including respiratory disorders. Toxicity is a significant health risk when working with unconventional materials. Fumes, particles and debris can enter the body by inhalation or by hand or mouth contact.

Chapter 9: Jewellery

Jewellery means ornaments which are made of valuable metals. Gold, silver, platinum, copper, brass, bronze, nickel and nickel silver are the metals which are used in jewellery or ornament making. Some of the common metals are:

Pure gold (Au) is soft, malleable and rich yellow in colour, but pure gold is too soft to make jewellery. For workability, the soft gold is usually hardened by mixing with other metals. The unit of measurement of gold is the carat. 18-carat gold means 75% gold; 24-carat gold means 100% gold. However, among all metals gold is top of the list in resisting corrosion and for its tarnish-resistant properties.

Silver (Ag) is a white metal which is soft, malleable and resists corrosion, but tarnishes when exposed to air or damp. Sometimes silver is alloyed with copper and it is then called sterling silver, though jewellery can also be made from silver alone.

Platinum (Pt) is a gray-white metal and is harder and heavier than gold. Its durability and malleability, and its colour and bright shine, enable jewellers to make fine jewellery. Sometimes platinum is used as a setting for gemstones. Platinum is without doubt the most precious metal and is expensive for jewellery making.

Copper (Cu) is a reddish-brown metal and is soft, malleable and corrosion-resistant, but tarnishes easily. Its attractive colour, easy workability and high melting point can make it rich material for jewellery.

Ornaments made of brass and bronze are also available on the market. Both are inexpensive alloys which are used in jewellery making. Brass is composed of copper and zinc; bronze contains copper and tin. So, the properties of the metal are important, and so are the right tools, equipment, techniques and processes required to cut, shape and join the various types of metals.

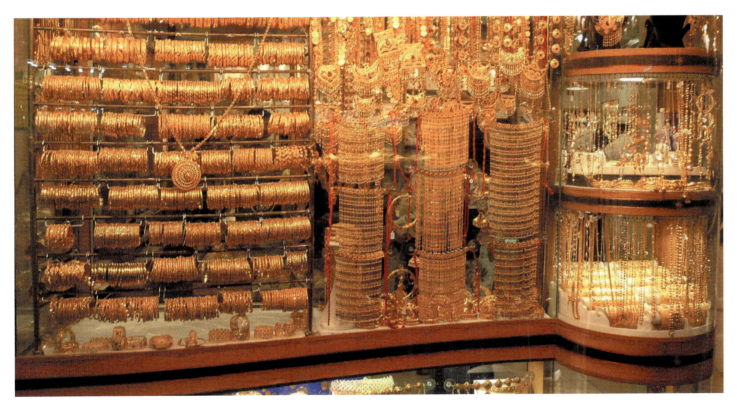

Jewellery (Gold Souk, Dubai)

Gold, silver and platinum are the precious metals which are traditionally used by jewellers. Before people were able to shape metal, they made jewellery out of seeds, berries, shells, and the bones and teeth of animals. Next came stone jewellery with the arts of carving and drilling technique. Hence it is evident that jewellery wearing has existed since the earliest phases of human existence. When people learned to work with metals, gold was the principal metal used for jewellery in the ancient world. Sumeria, Egypt, Nubia, Anatolia and Arabia are the countries where the earliest gold jewellery is found. In the modern world, Dubai is one of the cities in the Middle East where gold is sold in the open market. The market is called the Gold Souk: here large quantities of 24-carat gold jewellery in many varieties, shapes and qualities are available; moreover gold bars (or 'biscuits') – not to mention ATM machines for buying gold bars – are easily available, attracting many visitors.

The techniques, tools and processes depend on the type of jewellery that the jewellers make. The most common ornamental objects that jewellers produce are rings, ear-rings, chains, necklaces, pendants, bangles, bracelets, brooches and so on.

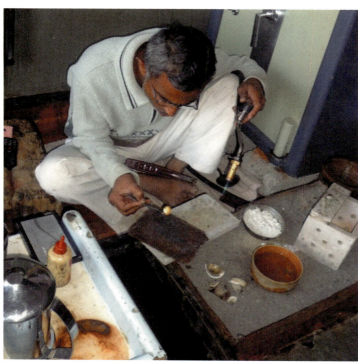

Traditional jewellery making (India)

Jewellers usually work at a workbench, and the common tools that they use are pegs, pliers, nippers, cutters, scissors, shears, tweezers, saws, soldering torches and tools, files, drills, hammers, mallets, tongs, polishing materials etc. For a special shape and design, jewellers rely on the casting technique. This is the technique by which the molten metal is shaped using a special tool and equipment. However, the basic steps for making ordinary jewellery are:

1.   *Select materials*: the first thing is to decide what types of metals the jeweller is going to use, and purchase accordingly. Most come in the form of sheet metal or wire. The sheet metals are available in various lengths, shapes, sizes and thicknesses. Wire comes in various shapes including full or half round, flat, square, oval and triangle. However, some jewellers make their own sheets and wire by recycling their own scrap cuttings, broken jewellery etc. To do this they first make ingot moulds from molten metal. Once cooled, the metal is removed from the mould and then the sheets or wire are made by hammering, rolling and stretching or passing through a series of grooves in the mill's roller.

2.   *Shaping and cutting*: this depends on what types of jewellery the jeweller is going to produce. For example, to create a ring, a jeweller has to measure the correct size and cut the desired length using a saw. Shaping and bending are done by hand or using pliers with moderate force. During sawing, the choice of an appropriate saw blade and the direction of the teeth while cutting are both important.

3.   *Soldering*: this is the process by which two ends of metal are joined together. A small piece of solder is cut from the metal sheet; the metal and solder are then cleaned using a pickling solution. The chips of solder are then warmed up slowly until a honey-like flux appears; with further heating the solder is allowed to flow. After soldering, the piece is allowed to cool and then put into

the pickle pot using copper tongs. After about five minutes the piece is taken out, rinsed and dried.

4.   *Drilling*: jewellery-making drills are mostly flexible-shaft, rotary or twist drills which are driven by a small electric motor; they come with drill bits of various sizes. There are also other drills which come with a foot pedal or other speed-regulating device. While drilling, technique is important, i.e. one must drill with appropriate pressure and speed, and insert a drill bit which is one size smaller than the desired hole.

5.   *Filing*: this process involves cleaning or clearing or removing burrs, ridges, scales etc., prior to carrying out the finishing process. Flat files, round or half-round files, triangular, square or round needle files are the types of files which are used for filing inside and outside, or in carving designs.

6.   *Finishing*: the first step is sanding: sandpaper is used to remove scratches and marks. The next step is polishing. This is done by working with a buffing machine. A good finish reflects the great beauty of the jewel.

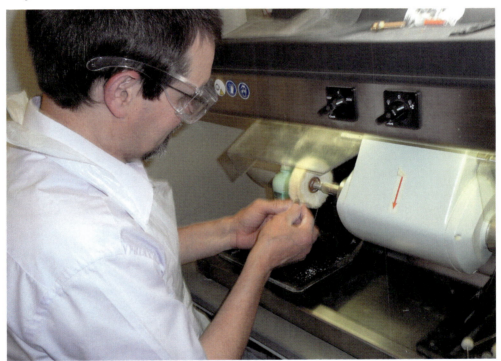

A buffing machine

WHAT ARE THE HEALTH ISSUES?

Major injuries are uncommon, but tool-related-accidents, and burns caused by molten metal or by chemical splashes (pickling solution), can occur. Noise, visual disorders and posture-related musculoskeletal disorders are not uncommon. Nickel-, cobalt-, chromium- and resin-related skin disorders (dermatitis) and cadmium-related respiratory symptoms and lung disorders have been seen amongst jewellers. Asthma, urticaria and hard-metal-related respiratory disorders have been found amongst jewellery polishers. Lead poisoning has been reported amongst silver jewellery makers. Increased incidence of lung cancer in jewellers has also been reported from New Zealand. It is important to always wear safety glasses when using a buffing machine. The machine usually has a hood and a filter system to minimise the debris that becomes airborne when polishing. During soldering or welding, emphasis must be given to wearing welder's goggles or safety glasses, gloves, mask, leather apron etc.

Chapter 10: Mosaics

Mosaic is an art form using small pieces of materials placed together to create decorative images or patterns. The various materials used to make mosaics are glass, ceramics, marble, stone, broken pottery, buttons, beads, bottle caps, mirror fragments, shells, pebbles and so on.

The first mosaics made of coloured stones, shells and ivory, dating back to the second half of the third millennium BC, were found in at Mesopotamia. Very early mosaics of basic patterns made of pebbles have also been discovered in Asia Minor and in the gardens of ancient China. The Ancient Greeks also used pebbles to create flooring. Mosaics, made by using 'tesserae', were first introduced in the fourth century BC. Tesserae were chunks of natural stone, cut into cubes. Tessera is a Latin word that means 'cube', and tesserae are usually made from various types of materials such as ceramic tiles, china, marble, glass etc. Mosaics have also been discovered in the excavated ruins of Pompeii.

Throughout civilisation, religion has played an important role in the development of the art of mosaic. Churches, synagogues and mosques were decorated with mosaics. Thus Christian mosaics in the fourth century, Jewish mosaics in the third to seventh century, and Islamic mosaics until the eighth century were flourishing and popular.

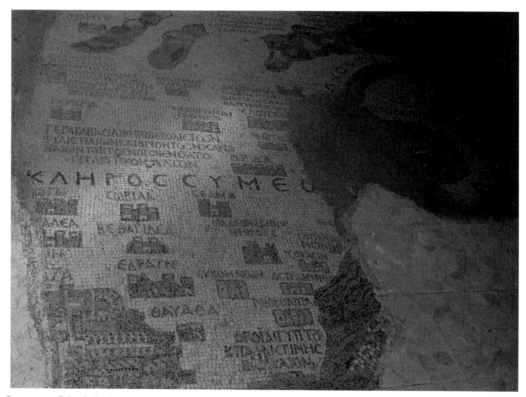

Mosaic art: Maldaba map (540-570) at the St.George Church, Madaba, Jordan

During the Renaissance period, as the technique improved and artisans travelled, mosaic art spread throughout the world. In the nineteenth century the birth of modern mosaics took place. However, almost everywhere in the twentieth century these arts were neglected. In the past few decades their popularity has been growing again due to increasing interest in decorative arts worldwide.

The surfaces or bases where mosaics are used as decoration are mainly cement floors, ceramic bases, glass surfaces, metal surfaces and wooden bases.

The tools and equipment which are needed are:

a) For designing: craft knife, marking pens, compasses, pencils, sketch book, ruler, graph paper, tracing paper, gummed brown paper.

b) For cutting and sticking: glue brush, tile scorer, glass cutter, tile cutters, mosaic nippers, hammer and hardie (chisel).

c) Glues and adhesives: cement, grout, epoxy resin, glue, paste.

d) For grouting: bowl, flat trowel, grout spreader, squeegee, palette knife, trowel, bucket or plastic container.

e) For cleaning: cloths, sponge, nailbrush, sandpaper, diluted hydrochloric acid.

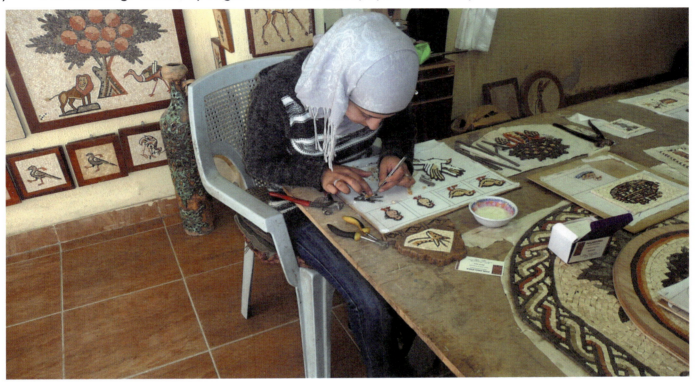

The art of mosaic making

The process of making mosaic arts can be varied but basic steps generally are

Step 1:   Prepare the base or surface.
Step 2:   Plan the design.
Step 3:   Select the material and prepare the tesserae by cutting and shaping.
Step 4:   Arrange and lay the tesserae.
Step 5:   Glue the tesserae in place.
Step 6:   Grout the mosaic.
Step 7:   Clean the mosaic.

WHAT ARE THE HEALTH ISSUES?

Tool- and material-related eye, face, and hand injuries can occur, especially from the 'tessera' chips. Cramp, twisting injuries and other upper limb disorders can also occur. Skin disorders (contact dermatitis) related to epoxy resin, glue and hydrochloric acid are seen. Special precautions must be taken while handling epoxy resins, whose toxic effects may include asthma, rhinitis, dermatitis and certain cancers (lungs, pancreas). Respiratory disorders, including mosaic-related dust disease (silicosis), have been reported. Emphasis must be given to personal protection in the form of safety glasses, goggles, mask, gloves, apron etc. during mosaic work.

Chapter 11: Musical instruments

A musical instrument is a device or object that produces sound. Sound is transmitted by vibration. The history of musical instruments goes back to the beginning of human culture and many earlier instruments are made of animal skin, bone, shell and wood. Ancient peoples used musical instruments such as drums, conch shell, trumpets etc. for hunting, rituals and religious ceremonies. The drum is most probably the first instrument made by humans, but the flute has also been in existence since prehistoric times, dating back to 67,000 to 37,000 years ago. Over the years, musical instruments underwent evolution as well as new inventions.

Basically, they are classified into three groups: a) *stringed instruments,* b) *percussion instruments* and c) *wind instruments*.

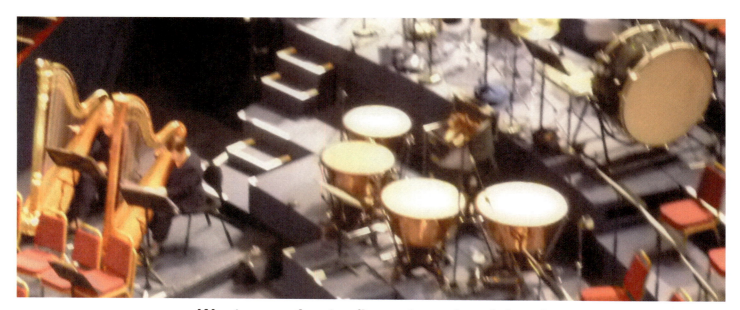

Western orchestra (harp, typani and drum)

a)   *Stringed instruments* have strings that are stretched across a wooden frame; they are usually made of steel, hair, gut (sheep's intestines) or nylon. The sounds of the vibrating strings are amplified by a sound bowl, which may be made from a naturally hollow object such as a gourd or turtle shell, or constructed as a wooden box. The guitar, violin, harp, cello, double bass and viola are stringed musical instruments that are usually part of the western orchestra. In South Asia, the main stringed instruments are the sitar, sarode, tanpura, esraj, surbahar, sursingha, dhothra, and violin, whereas in the Middle East, the stringed instruments are the oud and the quoun. However, to make any stringed instrument generally involves selecting, sawing and gluing various wood pieces. After assembling the various components, including wood pieces, sound box or bowl, strings and polish, numerous adjustments are necessary when fitting the strings to optimise the total character of the instrument and its playability. To make a stringed instrument some of the basic materials that are required are wood, a natural sound bowl (gourd), string, glue, sealer, lacquer, varnish or polish, and decorative materials. Sometimes finished wooden instruments, such as violins and sitars, are hung up for a period so that exposure to sunlight makes the wood darken. Varnish is a coating consisting of resins which may be natural or man-made. Coloured varnish is made by adding pigments or dyes. Some instruments are also inlaid with decorative materials such as wood, metal (gold) or plastic. The tools which are used depend on the type of stringed instrument one is making. However, some of the tool types are hand-working and carving tools, planes, chisels, gouges, knives, saws, scrapers, callipers, groove cutter, peg hole reamer, clamps, bending iron etc.

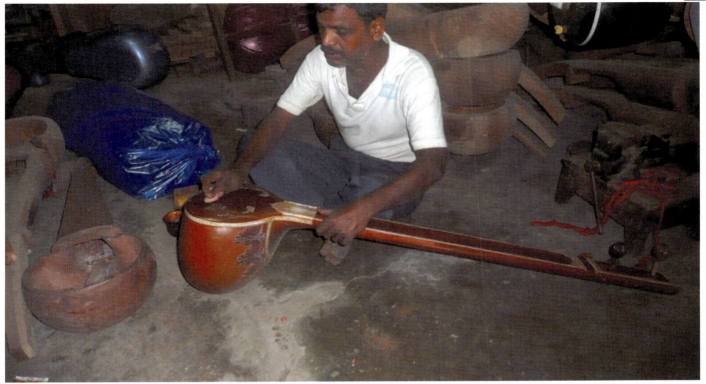

Sitar making (Indian string instrument)

b)   *Percussion instruments* are musical instruments that are played by hand, or sounded by being struck by beaters or struck against other, similar instruments. Beaters are usually wooden sticks, wire brushes or padded wooden mallets. African drums, Western orchestra tympani and drums, Egyptian or South Asian tablas, dholaks (Indian), xylophones, cymbals, clicking sticks and triangles are instruments which are in this group. Keyboard instruments such as the celesta, piano and harmonium (South Asia) also fall into this group, as they are played by percussion reeds although they are a kind of wind instrument. In drums the sound is usually produced by the wood as well as by the vibration of the stretched membrane. Different types of wood produce different types of sound. The greatest range and volume are produced when the wood is completely hollowed and covered with a membrane. Thus the drum has two basic components: the head and the shell. The head is the percussive surface of the drum and consists of one or both ends covered by a membrane made of animal skin such as goat, lamb or cow skin. Nowadays animal skins are mostly replaced by synthetic or plastic materials, usually polyester (polyethylene terephthalate). The shell is made of wood, and common woods are maple, birch, poplar and mahogany. Although drums exist in a wide variety of shape and sizes, the bowl and the tube are considered to be basic shapes. Some drum shells are made of metal such as steel, aluminium or brass, or of hard plastics or ceramics. Other accessories are straps made of leather, plastic or cloth; stands, made of steel or aluminium; rope, string, wooden pegs and drum hardware (metal) that are used to clamp, pull or adjust the drums or shell. African drums have rims made of metal or wood. The South Asian tabla has a black raised area made of rice, glue, graphite and iron filings.

c)   *Wind instruments* (brass and woodwind) are played by blowing down a hollow tube. As the length of the tube down which the air vibrates dictates the pitch, a number of different notes are possible if holes, which can be opened or stopped by the fingers, are drilled at intervals along the length. The main brass and woodwind instruments are the bugle, bassoon, clarinet, flute, French horn, oboe, piccolo, recorder, shehnai, trumpet and tuba.

30 The flute is the most common wind instrument, the one that is used in more cultures of the world than any other. Flutes can be made of bamboo, wood, metal or plastic (PVC). The bamboo flute consists of a cylindrical bamboo pipe that has a big hole (mouthpiece) for blowing air and six uniform holes which are covered by the movement of the fingers while playing. To make a wooden flute, one has to design it and choose the type of wood (usually softwood), and cut the wood to the correct size. After hand-carving the wood, a mark is made where the bore is to go and the finger holes are made by drilling, using a hand drilling machine. In case of a native American flute, parts like the flute tubing with holes, roost, plug, mouthpiece and bird are made separately and then joined

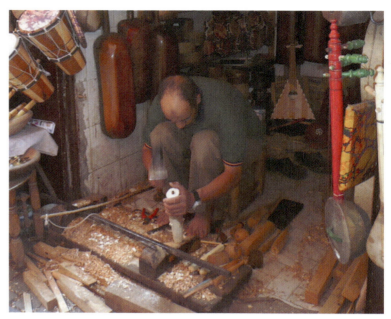

Flute making (North Africa)

together using glue, tape and lace. The tools which are used are the electric drill, hand counter, sink, dowelling, box cutter knife, seizers, v-jig and clamp.

Most flutes are made of metal and the modern method of flute making is by die casting, where molten metal is forced under pressure into steel dies. A group of connected keys may be made in one piece, or individual keys may be stamped out by a heavy stamping machine and then trimmed. The keys are fitted with pads made of cork and felt. Tone holes are made in the body of the flute by a process of pulling and rolling, or by cutting and soldering. The rods that support the keys are usually soldered to the body of the flute; pins and screws made of steel are used to attach the keys to the rods. Springs made of steel, bronze or gold are attached to provide tension in order to hold the cork and felt pads against the tone holes. The mouthpiece is then shaped and soldered to the head joint. The head joint, body and foot joint are fitted together and adjusted. After the flute has been tested for sound quality, the final stage involves cleaning, polishing and packing.

WHAT ARE THE HEALTH ISSUES?

Tool-related or manual-handling-related pain, discomfort or injuries are common. Noise hazards and posture-related musculoskeletal disorders can occur. Woodwork-related hand injuries and cases of string injuries have been seen. Infection can be contracted from animal hides: anthrax has been reported amongst African drum makers. Dust- and fume-related health issues are mainly from wood, metal and plastic materials. There is some risk of wood- or timber-related skin (primary irritant and contact dermatitis), eye and respiratory disorders (irritant or allergic) and wood-dust-related nasal cancers. Metal-related health issues arise from metal die casting, cutting, shaping, soldering etc., and the risks include respiratory, skin and eye disorders and certain cancers. Health issues relating to solvents, glue, lacquer, sealer, varnish (resin, pigments, dyes), polish, decorative materials (wood, plastic, gold) include skin disorders (dermatitis), respiratory disorders and carcinogenic risk. In many places, especially in developing countries, the habit of wearing protective equipment while working on musical instruments is lacking, and regular emphasis has to be given to education and self-protection.

Printing is a process for reproducing a subject (text, image, design or illustration) on a substrate, using ink. The substrate is the material that is printed on, such as paper, cardboard, vellum etc. The device that carries the linked image to the substrate is called an image carrier.
Printing can be done in two ways:

A)   *Impact printing*, by which the print subject is generated on an intermediate surface and then transferred on to paper. Letterpresses, lithography, and gravure/photogravure are types of impact printing. The basic differences between these three are: a) in letterpress, which is the oldest type of printing process, the printing surface is raised and lead is used for the image carrier; b) in lithography, the printing surface is flat and the image carrier is aluminium, paper or polyester; c) in gravure the image carrier is copper/chrome plated, the printing surface is recessed, and the surplus ink is scraped off using a doctor's knife or blade.

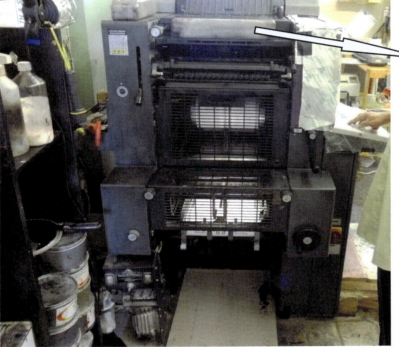

Image carrier

Litho printing machine

B)   Non-impact printing, by which an image is achieved without contact between the print mechanism and the paper. Examples are laser printing, thermal printing, ink-jet printing etc. Laser printing is a digital printing process whereby a laser beam is passed over a charged drum. The drum then collects the charged toner and transfers the image to the paper. Thermal printing is also digital printing: it produces a printed image by selectively heating a thermal paper which is coated with a chemical that changes colour when exposed to heat. Ink-jet printing is a kind of computer printing process whereby a digital image is created by propelling ink droplets on to paper, plastic etc.

The earliest form of printing was woodblock printing, which was being done in China before 220 AD, and in Egypt in the fourth century. The world's first printing technology featuring movable type was invented by a Chinese printer, Bi Sheng, in about 1040. However, the invention of the printing press, and of an improved movable type of mechanical printing technology, is credited to a German printer, Johann Genfleisch zum Gutenberg, in 1456. He used a letterpress method; the lithography technique first appeared in 1796. In the nineteenth century, the steam-powered rotary press replaced the hand-operated one. In 1875 offset printing, and in 1986 hot-metal typesetting were introduced into the printing process. Over the past four decades there have been tremendous advances in printing technology, especially the field of computer and digital printing. Phototypesetting in the 1960s, laser printing in 1969, thermal printing in 1972, ink-jet printing in

1976, 3D printing in 1984, X Gidee in 1991, and the digital press in 1993, are some of such inventions.

The printing process can be divided into three distinct steps or stages:

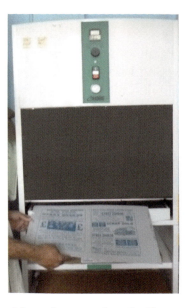

Non-impact printing

1. *Pre-printing stage*: preparing, composing or designing the printing job on the computer and then converting it into the printable format and finally into the image carrier.

2. *Printing stage*: this is the process of transferring the image to the substrate. The printing press is a power-operated machine that transfers text and images through contact with various types of inked surfaces on to paper or other material fed into the machine. The mechanism is such that the ink is applied to the printing surface and the printing is done by pressing the printing surface against the paper. In the litho printing technique, the lithographic ink is usually applied to the printing (image) area (wetted by ink), leaving the non-printing (image) area without any ink (wetted by water). In this type of printing machine, the alignment, paper movement (into and out of the machine), etc. are all automatic. In offset printing, the printing machine has three components:
   i) the in-feed, to feed the paper; ii) the printing unit; iii) the delivery, i.e. the printed sheet goes on to the pile.

3. *Post-printing stage*: this involves laminating, varnishing and finishing, including folding, cutting, stitching and binding. Finally come packaging and delivery.
In printing technology the common materials that are used are:
   a) papers, including colour, art and glossy,
   b) inks, including litho inks, UV cured inks and colour inks, and water. The ink may be fluid or solid; it may contain ingredients such as driers and other compounds,
   c) chemicals, including lacquers, adhesive solvents, n-hexane, toluene, and cleaning materials including acid and alkali,
   d) powder sprays (fine powder).

WHAT ARE THE HEALTH ISSUES?

Physical hazards are mostly due to manual handling, slips and trips and machinery-related accidents. Noise-related health issues include hearing impairment. Printer's asthma, toner allergy and printer ink allergy are conditions which may affect the respiratory tract, eyes and skin of the printing worker. There is a risk of lung cancer, bladder cancer and non-Hodgkin's lymphoma in the printing industry. Corrosive acids and alkalis can cause skin burns and eye damage, especially amongst plate developers. Solvents and inks can irritate the skin and can cause dermatitis. Some solvent vapour can cause dizziness and drowsiness, and can affect the central nervous system. Some solvents can, after prolonged exposure, cause damage to the liver, kidneys and other internal organs. There is a risk of toluene-related respiratory tract cancer, and dysfunction of the central nervous system cannot be ruled out. The Ultra Violet (UV) in UV inks and laminating adhesive can cause skin allergy and asthma (occupational). Some UV cured inks can cause skin cancer and risk to an unborn child. N-hexane neuropathy (peripheral neuropathy) has been reported.
To prevent health problems, the focus must be put on hand care, education, protective equipment and ventilation. Process automation, guarded machines or enclosure of machines and minimisation of leaks and spills are all important.

Chapter 13: Salt

Salt is sodium chloride (NaCl) in the form of cubic crystals that are used
a)   as a food supplement and in food processing,
b)   to remove snow and ice from the roads,
c)   in the chemical industry to produce chlorine,
d)   to stabilise soil in the construction industry,
e)   to soften water.

The earliest method of salt making was solar evaporation, i.e. the evaporation of sea water by the heat of the sun. This method is still in use, especially in hot, arid regions of the world, and near oceans, seas or salty lakes. In places where the climate did not allow solar evaporation, salt was produced by boiling salt water. This was done by pouring the salt water on to heated rocks or burning wood. Pans made of lead or iron were also used to boil water. This has now been replaced by a device known as a multiple-effect vacuum evaporator.

Quarrying is another method of salt production, and this is done either by quarrying exposed masses of rock salt (e.g. salt block mining in the Danakil depression) or by underground mining of salt deposits. Large rock salt deposits are found in the USA, Canada, Germany, Eastern Europe and China. The process of mining underground salt deposits involves undercutting and blasting.

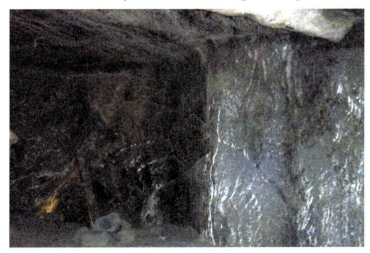

Rock salt face in a underground salt mine in Poland

To cut a slot, usually the gigantic chain saw is used and for blasting, initially a series of holes are made using electric drills, explosives (dynamite) are inserted, and the rocks are blasted. The blasted rocks are transported to crushing areas where crushing machines are used to reduce the size of the salt particles. Foreign particles are removed from the salt by a process called picking, whereby metals are removed by magnets and other materials by hand. If smaller particles are needed, the salt is pressed through a grinder consisting of two metal cylinders rolling against each other. Finally the crushed salt is passed though the screens to sort it by size, packed in bags and despatched to the consumer.

Water which contains a high concentration of salt is called brine, and the usual sources are oceans, seas and their backwater lagoons and pools, sea salt pans, salt marshes, underground salt water pools and hypersaline lakes. The traditional and conventional method of making salt is salt framing. Salt is concentrated in highly saline water near the coast, and salt crystals are produced by the solar evaporation. In the first instance, a salt field is prepared by creating a number of evaporation pans; simultaneously a well is dug out in one of the pans which fills with saline ground water. From the well, the saline water is usually transferred from one pan to the other through narrow channels.

 A wooden rib or wooden industrial broom is used to prepare the field. The salt water is dried up under the harsh sun, which transforms it into salt; sometimes polythene sheeting is used to improve quality. The entire process is done manually – in some places, by working with bare hands and feet. A salt mound is got ready to be transferred for further processing such as washing, crushing, refining and packaging.

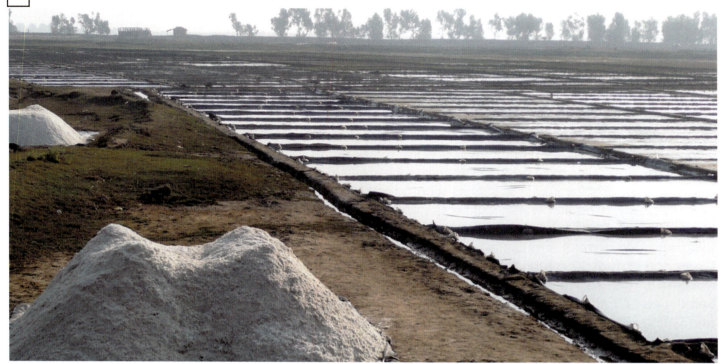

Evaporation pans and salt mound

Another way of manufacturing salt from brine is to use the multiple-effect vacuum evaporator method. Natural brines contain other substances such as magnesium chloride, magnesium sulphate, calcium sulphate, potassium chloride, magnesium bromide and calcium carbonate. Initially, the brine is treated chemically to remove the calcium and magnesium compounds, and then passed through the device consisting of three or more metal cylinders with conical bottoms. The brine in the first cylinder passes through the tubes, which are heated by steam. The brine boils and the steam enters the next cylinder, where it heats the brine there. The steam from this brine then heats the next cylinder and so on. Steam condensation takes place in each cylinder and the salt is removed from the bottom of the cylinder as a thick slurry. This is then filtered, dried and passed through screens in order to sort out the salt particles by size. Finally the salt is packed in bags or boxes.

WHAT ARE THE HEALTH ISSUES?

Fatigue and thermal strain, including heat exhaustion, heat cramps and skin rash, are caused by natural heat as well as working in hot salt mines or salt production works. Hand- and foot-related skin problems, including foot and hand irritation, traumatic ulcers, dermatitis, fissures, hyperkeratosis, callosities and mycotic lesions, are largely due to working with bare feet and hands. Therefore hand and foot protection, in the form of gloves and boots, is important. High incidences of caries and other periodontal diseases have been reported amongst salt-mine workers. Eye symptoms and eye disorders are prevalent in the form of eye irritation, reddening eyes, conjunctivitis, defective vision, cataracts and pterygium, and are due to irritation by direct sunlight and the glare caused by sunlight reflecting from salt crystals or brine, as well as irritation caused by fine salt particles in the working atmosphere. To prevent eye lesions, protective glasses must be used. Hypertension, muscular and joint pain, and other non-specific symptoms (giddiness, headache etc.) have also been reported. Risks of noise-induced deafness, hand vibration syndrome, and dust-related respiratory disorders are associated with underground salt mine extraction and salt-crushing processes. The commonest respiratory symptoms are coughs, phlegm and breathlessness.

Spices are vegetable products which are used as food additives, colourings and preservatives, in cosmetics and perfumes, and as herbal medicine. Humans have used spices since 50,000 BC; archaeological evidence of spice use (burnt cloves) has been found on kitchen floors at the Mesopotamian site of Terqa (Syria), dating back to 1700 BC. Cloves are mentioned in the Indian epic of *Ramayana*, and the Romans also used cloves in the first century BC. Cardamom was probably first used around 700 AD. It is mentioned in Indian medicinal literature, under the name *Charak Samhita*, between the second century BC and the second century AD. The use of spices in herbal medicine is traceable in India, China and Korea around 1000 BC. The Egyptians also used herbs in embalming.

The spice route played an important role in the development of the spice trade. Nutmeg originated in Indonesia, and Indonesian merchants took it to China, India, the Middle East and the east coast of Africa. The spice trade developed in the Middle East around 2000 BC, carried on mainly by Arab merchants who took it through India and the Middle East. Alexandria, in Egypt, was the main trading centre. This spice route, however, was land-locked, and was eventually replaced by the sea route: the monsoon winds helped the Arabs to sail from the spice-growing regions of the East to the Western European market. During the Middle Ages, spices such as black pepper, cinnamon, cumin, nutmeg, ginger, cloves and saffron were among the most sought-after and expensive products available in Europe. The plantations were in Asia and Africa. From the eighth to the fifteenth century, the Italian city of Venice acquired a monopoly of the spice trade, but after Vasco da Gama sailed to India in 1497 and discovered the new sea route to India, Portuguese sailors brought spices to Europe via Lisbon and thus the Portuguese succeeded to a growing monopoly of the spice trade. Christopher Columbus' discovery of the 'new world' ushered in new types of spices such as allspice, bell chilli peppers, vanilla and chocolate.

Currently many countries produce spices. In 2009-2010 the biggest producer was India (70%), followed by Bangladesh (9%), Turkey (5-7%), China (5.5%) and Pakistan (3%). Spices are available in the form of fresh, whole dried, pre-ground dried or ground. Whole dried spices have maximum shelf life of two years; that of ground spice is about six months. The flavour of spices depends on compounds that oxidise or evaporate when exposed to air. Grinding spices greatly increases their surface area and so accelerates oxidation and evaporation. To grind whole spice, a mortar and pestle are used.

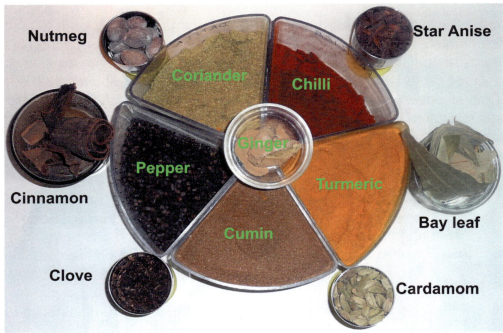

Some common spices

Various types of graters and grinders are also used, depending on the amounts to be processed. Many spices are soluble in oil or fat, so both are used during grinding. In these days of mass production, large quantities of spices are ground and packaged in factories or mills.

Some of the common spices are:

Cardamom: this is the fruit of the cardamom plant, which is a tropical herb with dark-green leaves and a long flowering stalk. The fruits are pale green or yellowish in colour, elongated in shape. There are three types of cardamom: black (large), green (small) and white. The black and green are the most commonly used as spices. The plant is cultivated under large, shady trees at an elevation of 600–1,500 metres in warm, damp climates with temperatures of 10-35°C and distributed rainfall of around 1500 ml. It is native to India, but is now also grown in Nepal, Bhutan, Sri Lanka, Guatemala, Tanzania, Zanzibar, Thailand, Pakistan and Bangladesh. Cardamom seeds are generally sown in September and October. They are planted out in June–July, and the harvesting is done when the seeds of the topmost capsules turn brown. The spikes are harvested using special knives. The capsules are then separated from the harvested spikes and dried. Traditionally, in Sikkim (India) the large cardamom is cured in *bhatti*, i.e. the capsules are dried under direct heating so that the cardamom comes in contact with smoke, which turns the capsule darker brown or black and gives it a smoky smell. The cured capsules are usually rubbed through a wire mesh for cleaning and removal of the calyx (tail). They are then graded, packaged and stored.

Cinnamon: this is the inner bark of a tropical evergreen tree which is harvested in the wet season, by cutting the shoots near the ground. This is done once in every two years. Using a semicircular blade, the shoots are first scraped and then rubbed with a brass brush to loosen the bark, which is split with a knife and peeled. The peels are overlapped one into another to form a quill. Quills are pieces of the inner bark that are curled into long rolls after drying. After 4-5 days of drying, the quills are rolled on a board to tighten the curls, and then placed in subdued sunlight for further drying. Finally they are bleached with sulphur dioxide, cut into strips and graded. Cinnamon trees are native to South-East Asia and now grow in India, Sri Lanka, Bangladesh, Java, Sumatra, the West Indies, Brazil, Madagascar and Zanzibar.

Cloves: these are the small brown flower buds of evergreen trees which can grow from seed to a height of 25-40 metres; they are planted in shady areas. The trees usually start to flower by the fifth year. The dried buds are picked by hand in both the summer and the winter season. One tree can produce around 30 kg of buds. Once picked, they are further dried in sunlight before being cleaned, graded and packaged. The length of cloves varies from half to three-fourths of an inch. The clove is a native of Indonesia, but is now cultivated in Indonesia, Zanzibar, Brazil, West Indies, Mauritius, Madagascar, India and Sri Lanka.

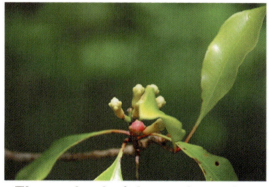

Flower buds (clove plantation, Zanzibar)

Pepper: the pepper plant is a perennial climber which has three types of runners: primary (the main stem), secondary and tertiary. The flowers, in clusters, grow only on the tertiary runners, opposite a leaf. The fruits are round berries. Each berry has a single seed, encapsulated in the flesh of the fruit. The berries are green at first, turning yellow and then red when fully ripe. It takes about nine months before the ripe berries are picked. The pepper is a tropical plant that grows in hot humid areas with high rainfall (2000 mm). It is native to India, but is also cultivated in Sri Lanka, Indonesia, Malaysia, Thailand, Brazil, Mexico, Madagascar and Tanzania. There are three types of pepper: white, black and green.

For white pepper, the berries are harvested when they are ripe or red and then boiled in water, or fermented, to remove the flesh. Then they are washed, cleaned, and dried in the sun for at least twelve hours, then sorted and packaged. For black pepper, the mature green berries are harvested and immersed in boiling water for a few minutes, which turns them black. They are then dried in the sun for 16-20 hours before being sorted and packaged. For green pepper, as soon as the berries are harvested they are separated, washed and conserved in brine (salt water, vinegar and citric acid).

Chilli: the chilli plant is bushy and grows up to two metres tall, but has weak branches which require support to prevent them drooping on the ground. It needs a warm climate, good sunlight and moist, well-drained soil, enriched with organic compost or fertiliser if necessary. The sowing time is April, and the chillies are harvested when the plant reaches the appropriate size and colour. Mature fruits give green chillies; fully ripe, red fruits give red chillies; or the fruits can be left on the bush until they shrivel up and dry. Chillies come in different sizes, shapes and colours, and the hotness also varies. Most are grown annually and sold in powder form.

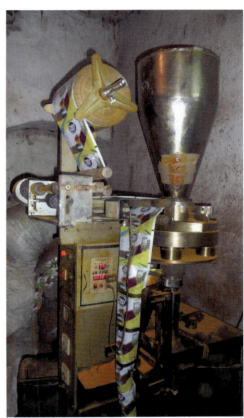

The freshly harvested chillies are first cleaned by hand, and then dried in the sun until they are crisp and ready to be ground by machine. Oil is sometimes used in the grinding process because the powder is soluble in oil. To obtain uniform mesh size, the powdered chillies are passed through sieves. Finally they are packed in polythene bags, which are heat-sealed by another machine. The chilli is a native of South America, but is now also grown in India, Sri Lanka, Bangladesh, Middle East, South Korea, China, Malaysia, Indonesia, Eastern Europe and the USA.

Turmeric: this is the dried rhizome of a plant that is cultivated in tropical and sub-tropical regions up to 1,500 metres above sea level (temperature about 20-30°C, rainfall above 1500 mm). India is a leading producer. Turmeric is usually sown in July and ready for harvesting in 7-9 months. It requires a rich soil; usually chemical fertilisers are used. After harvesting, the green rhizomes are boiled for hours until they produce white fumes with a characteristic odour, and then sun-dried on a clean floor for 10-15 days. To ensure uniform drying they are stirred 3-4 times. When fully dried, the hardened turmeric rhizomes are crushed to powder in a spice-grinding machine, then packaged and sealed. Nowadays an automatic machine does all three processes (crushing, packaging and sealing) in one.

Spice grinding machine

WHAT ARE THE HEALTH ISSUES?

Harvest-related physical injuries include knife cuts and falls. Smoke damage and burns may occur. Spice cultivation can cause damage from handling chemicals in pesticides, herbicides and fertilisers. Hearing, eye, skin and respiratory hazards are associated with grinding, milling, blending or packaging various spices. Hearing loss can be caused by excessive noise during grinding. Dry chillies can irritate eyes and skin. If hot chilli powder gets into eyes it can cause blindness. Other eye symptoms are conjunctivitis, rhino-conjunctivitis and occulo-nasal trouble from dust. Skin troubles include pruritus, irritation, burning sensation, urticaria and allergic contact dermatitis. Spice dust can cause both irritant and allergic respiratory disorders. Acute and chronic respiratory symptoms include increased risk of asthma and chronic obstructive pulmonary disease.

Chapter 15: Stone crafts

Stone crafts involve stone carving. Various types of stones are used to make handicrafts, utensils, furniture, art objects, home decorations, sculptures, monuments and for construction work (building materials).

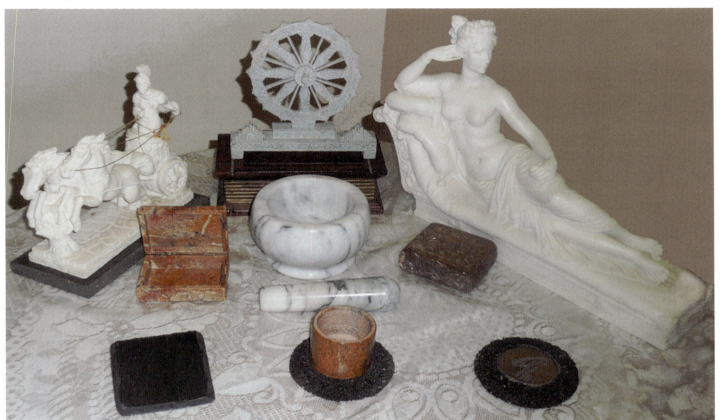

Stone crafts made of marble, alabaster, sandstone, granite, slate, volcanic rock and fossil stones

Back in the earliest stages of human existence, in prehistory, people created stone tools, weapons and artefacts from stone and rock fragments. Ancient civilisations such as the Egyptians, Indians, Greeks and Romans gave importance to stone work in creating monuments, temples, sculptures, buildings and other art works. In the modern world, besides traditional types, stone works are evolving new forms and ideas.

Materials for stone work are naturally available stones which are acquired by quarrying blocks, slabs or pieces from geological sources. Some stones are soft, some are hard and some are medium. Fossil stones are also used. All stones can be carved, but selection of stone depends on its colour and hardness as measured by the Mohs scale. The most common stones which are used are:

Marble is a metamorphic stone with hardness of 6. The colour is usually white, but green, black, blue, grey and olive coloured marbles are also available.

Alabaster is a soft, metamorphic stone with hardness varying between 2 and 3 and is available in a variety of colours such as beige, brown, cloud-grey, green/red, honey/tan, orange, white ,white and black, white and brown, yellow and so on.

Limestone (Chalk) is a medium type of sedimentary stone with hardness of 4 and is available mainly in buff or cream colour, but red, yellow, green brown and tinted black are also found.

Soapstone is a soft, metamorphic stone with hardness of 2. Usually the colour is black, but some soapstones are speckled with red, grey or yellow. Some are white with grey markings.

Slate is a metamorphic stone with a variation of hardness from soft to very hard.-on the basis of quartz - mica relation. The colour is usually black or grey, but green, red, brown and yellow are also found.

Sandstone is a medium stone from sedimentary rock with hardness of 4; the colour can be red, brown, grey, blue or black. The colour and hardness depend on the mineral content and the binding materials.

Granite is a hard stone from igneous rock with hardness of 8. The colour can be pink, white, grey, dark grey, black, blue-grey or blue-white.

Fossil stones are stones in which animals or plants have been fossilised and turned to stone. In the process of fossilisation the soft tissues of animals are broken down, while the hard parts like bone and teeth are buried and gradually mineralised. Some animals have been found frozen solid; and insects have been trapped in resin and hardened into stone. Plant fossils are from plant parts such as trunk, branches, leaves, roots, cones or seeds. Sometimes the plant materials have been replaced by minerals. Petrified wood also becomes stone. Some ornamental and decorative stones are formed from fossils. Amber fossil stones, Indian fossil stones, Brownwood fossil stones (USA), Mandra Bair fossil stones (Bulgaria) and Sinks fossil stones (Morocco) are some of the fossil stones with unique images that are excellent for stone crafts and as decorative building materials.

The process of stone carving begins with the *selection of the object* as well as the *selection of the stone.* The *selection of the object* largely depends on the idea and imagination of the artisan by which he or she creates his or her object. They may get ideas from their surroundings which they observe, as the world provides them with abundant materials. Some objects are necessary items, some are imaginative and some are art objects.

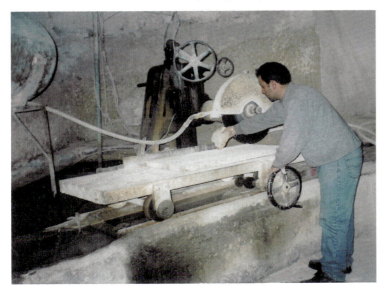

Stone sawing

Once the object is selected, the next step is the *selection of the stone*. This depends on the colour, hardness and size and weight of the stone which is suitable for making the particular object. Usually soft stones are preferred. Stones with cracks or faults are avoided.

Next comes the *carving of the stone*. For that a square or rectangular piece of stone is usually chosen. Prior to carving the stone, the carver may use sketches which are drawn or marked on the stone using pencil, chalk or crayon.

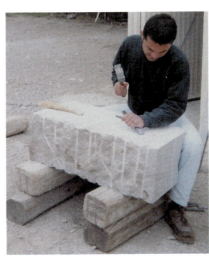

Roughing out by using chisel and hammer

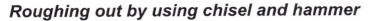

40   The next step is *roughing out*, which means knocking off the unwanted portion of the stone by using chisel, hammer, power tools (stone cutter, driller, grinder), etc.; the general shape of the object is made by using a toothed chisel or claw. A brush is used to remove the loose chips and small stones. To clean the stone, chemicals such as hydrofluoric acid or hydrochloric acid are used.

After this comes the *refining procedure*, which means smoothing the shape from rough to smooth: for this, tools such as straight-edge or cape chisels, rondels, rasps, files and rifflers are used. The final stage is further *smoothing, polishing and finishing*. Sandpaper, sand cloth, garnet paper, and waterproof silicone-carbide-coated paper (wet and dry carbide paper) are used to ensure a smooth and well-polished finish. Glossy polishing is done with tin oxide, iron oxide, stannic oxide or aluminium oxide. Diamond abrasives, muslin buffs, wheels with mandrels etc. are also used, especially for polishing the hard stones. Waxing is done by applying wax with a soft cloth. Finishing involves mounting (on a base), checking for cracks and fractures, and lastly packaging.

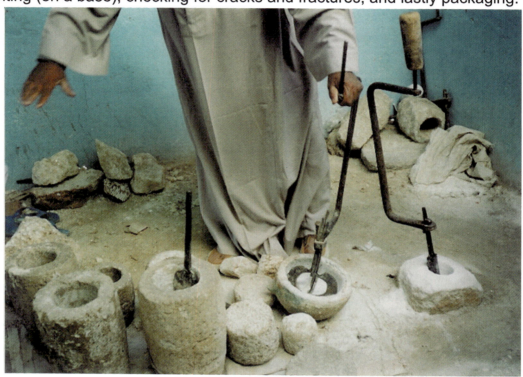

Traditional bowl making (Egypt)

WHAT ARE THE HEALTH ISSUES?

Stonecraft-related physical injuries can occur during manual handling, lifting or carrying or from slipping, tripping, falling or being hit by flying objects, i.e. stone chips. Safety glasses, face mask and goggles are necessary to prevent eye and face injuries from flying bits of stone. Always keep provision for eye wash, cotton wool and swabs. Amputation injuries during machine-operated stone-cutting work have been reported. Noise and hand-transmitted vibration can give rise to deafness and hand-vibration syndrome from using powered tools and pneumatic equipment. Ergonomic risk factors relating to manipulative dexterity, posture, vibration exposure and chipping hammers include musculoskeletal and locomotor disorders and upper limb disorders. Burns and contact dermatitis can occur from stone-cleaning materials such as hydrofluoric acid, hydrochloric acid etc. Silicosis, chronic obstructive pulmonary disease (COPD), tuberculosis and lung cancer are further stone-dust-related respiratory hazards or risk factors. Importance must be given to the dust mask, respirators, ventilation, exhaust system and provision of a vacuum cleaner at the workplace.

Textiles are made from fine fibres in the form of thread or yarn. The source of these fibres may be plant, animal or synthetic. Yarn is formed by spinning (twisting together) these fibres. Textiles are made by interlacing the yarn or thread by various methods, of which weaving and knitting are the most common. Nowadays this is done by modern textile machines, although weaving, spinning and knitting by hand are ancient arts and are still popular crafts.

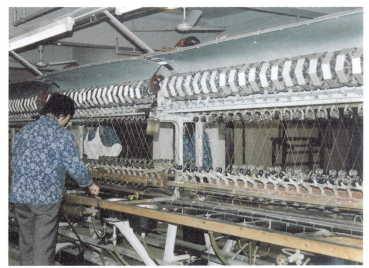

Textile machine weaving (silk) in China

In weaving two sets of threads or yarns are used: one set for lengthwise use and the other for side to side (crosswise) use. The crosswise (weft) thread is passed under and over a set of lengthwise (warp) threads. This way of weaving cloth is done by a weaving machine or device, called a loom. The use of looms goes back to 4000 BC and to the ancient Egyptians; the Chinese also used them. Knitting is another method by which cloth and other textiles are made. It is done by creating interlocking loops with various types of knitting needles. The knitting can be done by hand or by a knitting machine. The discovery of a decorated cotton sock in Egypt suggests that the knitting method was used in Egypt in the first millennium AD.

Like knitting, crochet is also a method of creating fabric from thread or yarn, this time by using a crochet hook; it is done by pulling loops of thread through other loops. The only differences between knitting and crochet are, first, that a crochet hook is used instead of knitting needles, and secondly, that in crochet, during the process of creating the fabric only one loop is active at a time.

Once the textile is made, it goes for bleaching, dyeing, colouring, printing and other finishing processes. The bleaching is done using various kinds of bleaches and various methods; it makes the fabric white, clean and dirt free.

Dyeing or colouring was originally done using plant products or dyes derived from insects. However, most dyes are now synthetically produced.

Coloured designs and printing are common textile arts. Designs can be created by weaving together fibres of different colours, as in tartan, or by adding colour stitches to the cloth, or by wax designs and dyeing (batik designs), or by wood-block printing on the cloth. After bleaching and colouring, the fabrics go for various treatment processes. The types of treatment are largely dependent upon the types of fibres used. For example, cotton and rayon shrink when they are washed. To prevent that, they have to be treated with an anti-shrink finish.

The textile-making fibres are:
Plant (vegetable) fibres: cotton, flax, jute, hemp and sisal fibres are used to make cloth and other textiles.

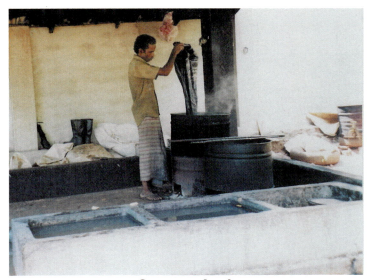

Cotton dyeing

Cotton fibres come from seeds. The boll of the cotton plant bursts when ripe and seeds are exposed within a white fluffy mass which is the cotton fibres. Most cotton grows in the warm, moist tropical and sub-tropical areas of the world such as America, India and Africa.

Flax comes from seeds, which grow in cool moist climates; the leading producing areas are Canada, Europe, China and India. The use of plant fibres (cotton, flax etc.) in textiles goes back to the fifth or fourth millennium BC in India and Egypt.

Jute: raw jute is an off-white coloured fibre that can be spun into a coarse, strong thread. It is ligno-cellulose fibre, i.e. partly wood and partly textile. Jute grows in warm and wet climates. Bangladesh and West Bengal in India are the most famous jute-growing areas of the world, where high temperature, high humidity and monsoons allow the jute fibres to develop.

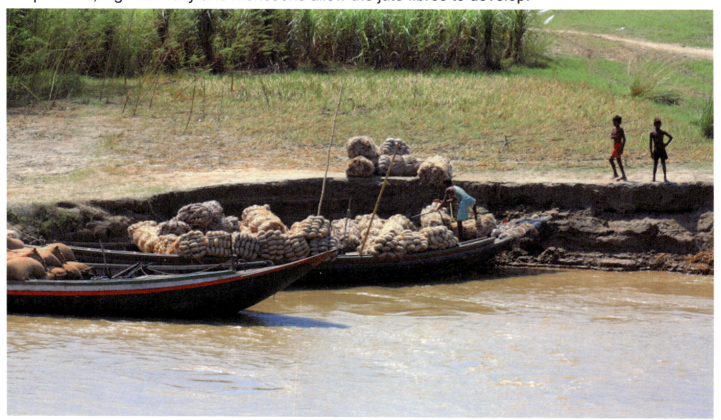

Jute fibre transfer to the mill

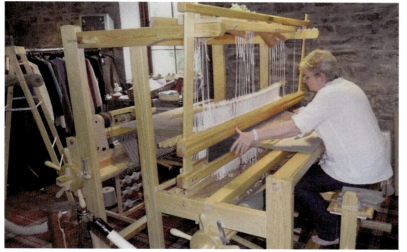

Animal fibres: these are mainly wool and silk. Wools are made from hair or fur from domestic goats or sheep. The most famous products are Shetland wool, Harris tweed, alpaca wool, lama wool, mohair and vicuña wool. Hair from the cashmere goat and the angora goat, camel hair and hair from the angora rabbit are used in the production of textiles, including coats, jackets, blankets and other warm coverings.

Shetland wool weaver

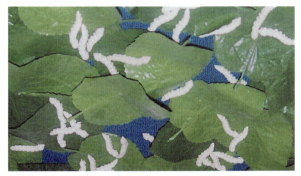

Silk worms on mulberry leaves

Wadmal is coarse, warm woollen cloth from sheep's wool, produced in Scandinavia, Iceland and the British Isles and dating back to the Neolithic period.

Silk comes from cocoons made by silkworms, which are the larvae (caterpillars) of silk-moths, feeding on mulberry leaves. A single cocoon is spun into a long, fine, smooth, shiny thread; and to make one metre of silk fabric requires 3000 cocoons. To acquire such a large quantity of silk fibres, the silkworms are farmed; this is known as sericulture.

The next process is *reeling*, which is putting the cocoons through hot and cold immersions so as to be able to unwind the cocoon. The cocoons float in the water as the fibres are rapidly wound on to wheels or drums. Reeled silk is transformed into silk yarn by a process called throwing before the silk is wound on to bobbins. The major silk-producing countries are China and India. Silk fibres were first developed in ancient China between 6000 and 3000 BC.

Synthetic fibres: nylon, acrylic, polyester and spandex are some of the man-made synthetic fibres which are produced from chemicals and are usually made by the method of polymerisation. They are mostly used in the production of clothing, and the fibres are much stronger than natural fibres. They are usually waterproof, easy to wash, crease-resistant and insect-resistant, which makes them suitable to wear as outer garments.

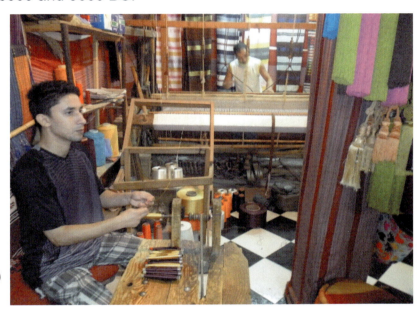

Bobbin loading and weaving (cotton, silk and synthetic fibre)

WHAT ARE THE HEALTH ISSUES?

Animal, vegetable and synthetic fibres can cause allergy, irritation and, although rare, anthrax has also been reported. Byssinosis is the textile workers' disease. Cotton, flax, soft hemp and sisal are the vegetable dusts which can cause byssinosis, whereas jute and some industrial hemp can cause non-specific airway irritation. Chronic bronchitis and chronic obstructive respiratory disorders are also prevalent amongst textile workers. Repetitive-work and posture-related back pain and other musculo-skeletal disorders, including trauma, have been reported, especially amongst women, as large number of women and children are employed in the textile industry in many countries. Risk of physical injuries including hand injuries, burns etc., and noise-induced hearing loss amongst textile factory workers, can occur. In the silk textile industry, dermatitis from handling the decomposition products of a parasite in the cocoon, respiratory allergies, and rhinitis are found. Increased risk of certain cancers (bladder, gastro-intestinal etc.) is prevalent amongst textile workers. Dyes can also cause allergy, irritation, asthma and dermatitis. Some dyes have carcinogenic effects and possibly other toxicity.

Chapter 17: Umbrella making

An umbrella is a device to protect a person from sun, rain and snow. The use of umbrellas has been recorded in ancient Africa, Asia and Europe and it was a common accessory amongst gods, goddesses, kings, queens, and noblemen and women. From the nineteenth century onwards it was popular amongst wealthy people, but now-a-days it is an essential item among most peoples of the world. Over the centuries the quality of umbrellas has changed; so has their mechanism. Once there were stick umbrellas; now we have collapsible ones. Umbrellas used to be made from cane, bamboo, whalebone or wood; nowadays they are more likely to be plastic, steel or other metals. Modern umbrellas are lighter, stronger and slimmer. There are two main types: straight and folding. The opening and closing mechanism can be manual or automatic. There are many varieties of umbrellas available, including fashion, automatic, anti-ultra violet, anti-static, luminous/reflective, water resistant or waterproof, water/oil repellent and so on.

An umbrella consists of a) handle, b) shaft, c) canopy, d) stretchers, c) ribs and f) runners. To make an umbrella all these parts have to be assembled; this is usually done by hand. The structure or frame is made first by assembling ribs, stretchers and shaft, after which a canopy is fitted.

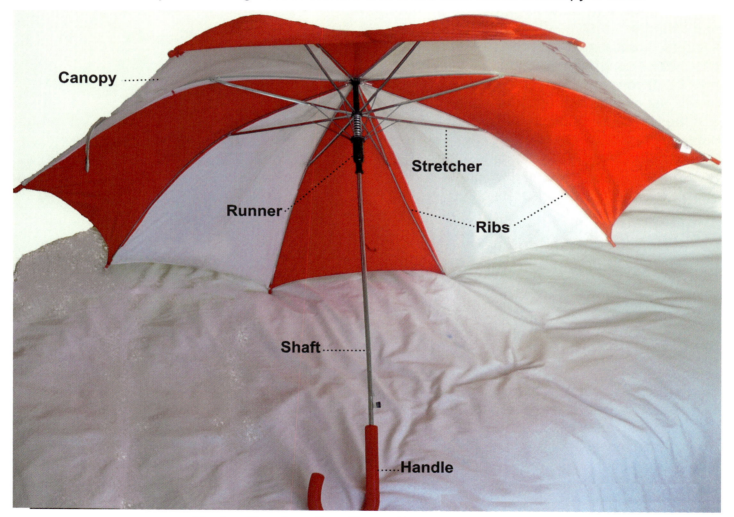

Umbrella showing its various components

The shaft, ribs, stretchers, runners and handles are usually made of wood, metal (steel, aluminium), plastic, carbon fibre or glass fibre whereas the canopy is made of fabric. There are various types of fabrics such as linen, cotton, silk, leather, polyamide/polyester, nylon taffeta or other waterproof fibres.

Microfibre fabrics with water-repellent finishes are also used. The choice of fabric depends on the manufacturer, bearing in mind its pattern, design, attractiveness, durability, lightness and waterproof properties. A wooden pattern and a sharp knife are used to cut the umbrella panels from the fabric. The canopy is hand-sewn in individual panels to the ribs. The ribs run under the canopy of the umbrella. The stretchers connect the ribs with the shaft of the umbrella.

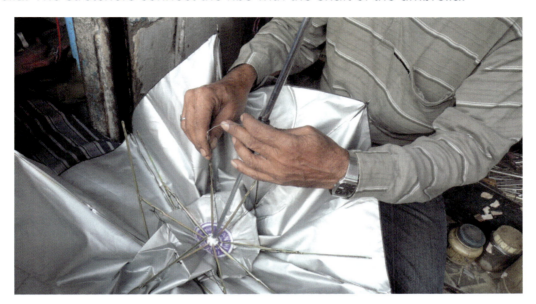

Assembling the ribs and stretchers

Each rib is attached to the shaft of the umbrella by fitting it into a top notch (a thin, round nylon or plastic piece with teeth around the edges), and a thin wire is used to hold it. Each stretcher is connected to the shaft with a plastic or a metal runner which moves along the shaft when the umbrella it is opened or closed. The ribs and stretchers are connected to each other with a joiner. The joiner is a small, jointed metal hinge which opens and closes as the umbrella is opened or closed. In the shaft of every umbrella, there are two catch springs (metal) which need to be pressed when the umbrella is slid down the shaft for closing. The catch springs are usually inserted in the metal shaft, but in case of a wood shaft, a space must be hollowed out. A pin or a blocking device is placed in the shaft above the upper catch. This will usually prevent the canopy from sliding past the top of the umbrella, if the runner goes beyond the upper catch spring. Lastly, the handle is connected to the shaft using screws or glue. Finally the umbrella is finished and packaged. Finishing also involves coating, printing and other fashionable touches.

WHAT ARE THE HEALTH ISSUES?

Injuries or accidents can be caused by various umbrella-making tools or parts such as wire, runners, catch springs, needles, pins, knives, scissors, rotary cutters, sewing machines etc. Injuries can occur from the sudden collapse of a frame. There is a risk of posture-related musculo-skeletal disorders, and of injury from twisting or dexterity movements. Eyestrain and eye disorders cannot be ignored. Materials (wood, metal, aluminium, carbon fibre, glass fibre etc.) can produce skin and respiratory disorders; fabric-related chemical sensitivities can cause lung, skin, liver and kidney lesions. Finishing- or coating-related chemical hazards can cause acute or chronic issues. Some of the chemicals are carcinogenic. Glues, resins and driers, mineral spirits or solvents and polybutene can cause dizziness, headache, nausea, eye trouble, respiratory disorders and skin irritation. Cancers and neurological disorders from overexposure to solvents cannot be ruled out. The wearing of personal protective clothing is important.

Chapter 18: Woodworking

Woodworking in the form of carving and turning is among the most traditional and skilled crafts throughout the world. Craftsmen have always made beautiful wooden items from trees. Over the years and throughout history their skilful hands have produced sticks, utensils, tableware, buckets, boxes, jewellery, combs, barrels, wheels, building materials and furniture, boats and other transport items, sports and game products, musical instruments, dolls and toys, weapons and so on. It is not known when woodworking first began, though its existence in the prehistoric period is undoubted. Wood was one of the first materials that early humans worked on. Among the early findings of wooden objects are sticks from the Kalambo Falls in Zambia and from Clacton-on-Sea in England, and also 400,000-year-old spears from Schöningen, Germany.

Wood comes from trees and trees consist of bark and wood. There are three types of woods: hardwoods, softwoods, and plywood or medium-density fibreboards (MDF). Hardwoods are from angiosperm plants which have got broad leaves and flowers; softwoods are from coniferous plants. Plywood and fibreboards are man-made. Hardwoods are mainly used in the construction and building industries and for furniture, utensils and fuel. Softwoods are used in the building, furniture, pulp, paper and print industries; plywood and fibreboard are used in the building industry (floors, roofs, walls), in scaffolding, furniture, packaging and boxes, sports goods, the internal body structure of vehicles, wind-breaking panels etc. Tropical trees are mostly hardwoods. Sometimes coconut shells, gourds or bamboo which are not really plants are used by woodworkers to manufacture bowls, spoons, containers and musical instruments, and in the construction or building industries.

Forestry and logging:
31% of the world's land area is forest. As the earth's population increases, the demand for wood, logs, timber is also increasing and thus forest areas and woodlands are decreasing. The question remains: are we doing enough by planting trees to make up for these losses?

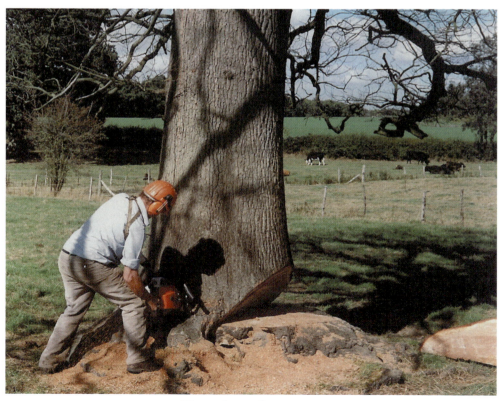

Tree logging

Logging is the process of cutting down the forest trees; clear-cutting is the harvesting method whereby all the standing tress are cut in a selected area. There are many different logging methods. To mention just a few: tree-length logging, full-tree logging, cut-to-length logging. Whatever method is used, the bucker turns trees into logs and the process of cutting a felled, de-limbed tree into logs is called bucking. Limbing is cutting off the remaining branches (usually from the trunk) of the felled tree. Chain-saws, harvesters (heavy foresting vehicles), skidders, forwarders etc. are used for felling, de-limbing and bucking trees. The logs are then transported to a sawmill to be cut into timber; the usual modes of transport are road (trucks or skeleton cars), river (timber rafting) or rail.

Timber and lumber:
A craftsman uses timber and lumber, which are made from tree trunks after stripping the bark and lopping the branches. Most timber is cut or split into planks and blocks prior to its use by craftsmen. Planks are made by splitting or sawing. Splitting is done using an axe or froe; sawing with a frame saw or pit saw. Nowadays, to obtain better quality planks, modern sawmills are used. Accurately cut planks are made with saws and the process is called 'milling'.

With modern machinery, various types of cuts are possible. Next step is seasoning, which means drying the wood. Drying can be done in two ways: either under the sun or in a kiln.

Wood grain and colour:
The term 'grain' refers to the way a tree grows in different seasons or in each year (growth rings). Craftsmen use the direction of the grain lines (along, against, across and end) to align the wood or for other woodwork techniques. The texture and density of the wood also play an important part in wood workability. Decorative effects, such wavy patterns in the wood, barks, swollen burrs or sprouts, are used as figuring.

Woodworkers also exploit various types of natural colour in the wood. The natural colour might be red, yellow, black, brown or mahogany; these are mostly hardwoods, but colourful softwoods are also available which are mostly reds.

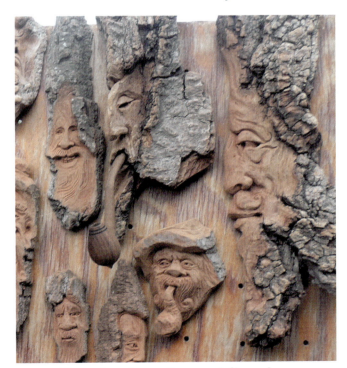

Tree bark and wood figuring

The colour depends on how the tree grows: soil type, water and the amount of sunshine. Sapwood is the youngest wood of the tree (the trunk), which is pale in colour; gradually the colour changes as it becomes heartwood. The growth rings of some trees also appear as different colours. Clearly, then, for various types of woodwork and carving, woodworkers use grain and colour in their creative techniques.

Woodworking:
The techniques involve designing, carving, and turning, shaping and joining the woods. Drawing or transferring a design on to wood is the first step in woodworking, and for that a sharp pencil, compasses, graph paper, photocopier, stencils etc. are needed. The craftsman then carves the block of solid wood into objects, which involves incising, cutting, stamping and various types of curving. Turning is the process by which the article is 'turned' for shaping or further curving.

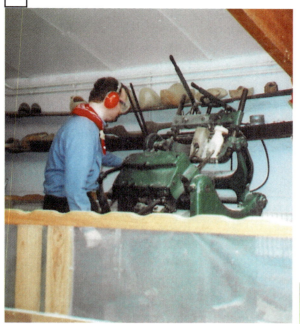

Joining is the technique by which two pieces of wood are connected together; the process involves edge-to-edge or end-to-end joining, or alternatively overlapping, or fastenings and fixings. For woodworking, the chief tools and equipment are axes, adzes, knives, hammers, chisels, gouges, planes, saws, drills and lathes. To hold the wood securely and prevent movement the craftsman uses vices, clamps, frame and jigs; to smooth an object the tools are scrapers, rasps, files, rifflers, abrasives and burnishers (sandpaper, bone, stone or metal) etc. For joinery work, the joiner uses glue, dowels, nails or wedges. Joiners also make slots and sockets, and to ensure a tight fit some joiners use mortise and tenon joints at the corners. Decorating and finishing is the final stage of woodworking.

Woodworking

Decorating involves colouring, figuring, veneering, parquetry, metallic finishes, and embellishment or inlay. For embellishment or inlay work, materials like metal, wire, shell, ivory (nowadays, plastic) and bone are used. Finishing work involves polishing, varnishing and painting. In these processes, oil, wax, resins, French polish, lacquer etc. are applied.

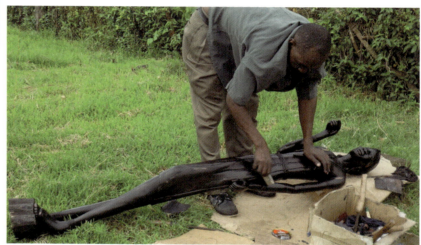

Figuring work (finishing), Kenya

WHAT ARE THE HEALTH ISSUES?

Physical injuries can occur during manual handling, lifting or carrying, or from slipping, tripping, falling or being hit by flying objects. Tool-related or machine-related injuries can also occur. Noise-induced hearing loss, and hand/arm vibration syndrome, are common occupational diseases amongst forestry workers, chain-saw workers, timber and lumber workers. Increased risk of musculo-skeletal and connective tissue disorders, as well as posture-related lower back pain, are also associated with the lumber and wood product industries. Woodworkers are at higher risk from certain cancers (nasal, ethmoid or paranasal sinuses, lung, stomach, liver, lymphatic and haemopoietic system etc.). These are due not only to the wood dust itself but also to chemicals that are applied to wood, including preservatives and other carcinogenic agents associated with woodwork. Other disorders associated with exposure to wood dust include occupational asthma, chronic obstructive lung disease, rhinitis, and conjunctivitis or rhino-conjunctivitis. Dermatitis and occupational skin diseases are also found in woodwork industries.

Chapter 19: Whisky making

Whisky is an alcoholic drink in the spirit group. The word 'whisky' is of Celtic origin and the drink is native to Scotland and Ireland. There is dispute as to where whisky was invented. The first written records of Scottish whisky making date back to 1494, although some claim that the drink was invented in Ireland about 1000 years ago and the art was then taken to Scotland by monks. Nowadays the whisky-making countries are Scotland, Ireland, USA, Canada, Japan, Europe, South Africa, India, Australia and the Far East. Most whiskies are made from cereal, except Indian whisky which is made from molasses. The main raw materials for whisky making are water, yeast and grain. The grains used are barley or malted barley or in combination with corn, wheat, oats or rye. To make whisky pure, cold water is important. In Scotland, most distillers rely on spring water, whereas in the USA they use hard limestone water with a high mineral content.

Aroma and flavour are important in whisky making. The influence of climate, geology, water, heather, sea breezes, seaweed, peat, charcoal, barley and other grains, copper and wood (oak barrel or cask) – all play a part in the aroma and flavouring of the whisky. In the whisky world, the famous four styles of whisky production are single malt whisky (Scotland), grain whisky (Scotland), Irish pot still (Ireland) and bourbon (USA). Here is the example of Scotland's single malt whisky production. It is made from the finest barley, and the following six steps are usually followed to produce it:

1.   *Malting*: malt is the result of a process whereby the cell walls of the barley break drown so that the starch contained in the barley is converted into sugar. Malting is done in three stages: steeping, germination and kilning. Steeping means soaking the barley grain in water in steeps (large vessels) so that the germination process can start.

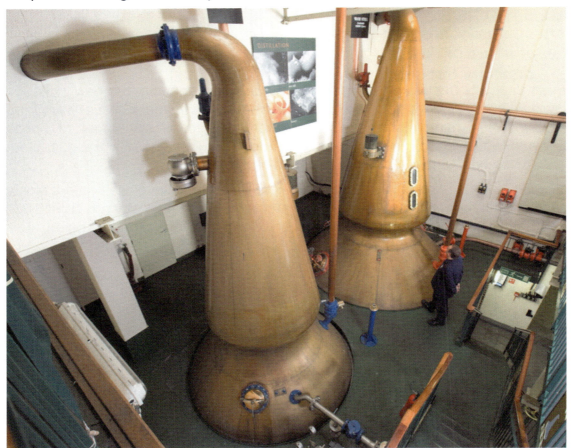

The copper still in the still house, Oban distillery Scotland

Water is added in 2–3 batches and oxygen is pumped in. Germination starts once the grain leaves the steep. It usually takes 24–36 hours to enable the grain to develop roots and shoots. After 5–9 days the germination process is stopped by drying in a kiln. During the kiln stage, the malt is 'peated'. It is the smoke of the peat fire which gives some whiskies their particular flavour.

2.   *Milling and massing*: the dry malted grain is crushed or ground into floor and is then called 'grist'. The grist is then mixed with hot water in the wash tun. The wash tun has a double bottom with thin perforations that let the sugar run off in a liquid form that is called 'wort'.

3.   *Fermentation*: the wort is cooled and then pumped into fermentation vessels where yeast is added. The action of the yeast is to convert sugar into alcohol and carbon dioxide. It takes 2–3 days for the fermentation process to complete and this fermented liquid is called 'wash'. It usually contains 8–9% alcohol.

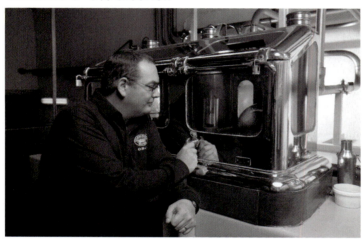

Distillery operator checking the gravity and temperature of the spirit, Oban distillery Scotland

4.   *Distillation*: in the production of malt whisky, the wash is distilled twice. The pot still is the traditional method of distilling malt whisky. It is made of copper; the shape and size varies from distillery to distillery.

The shape of the pot still significantly affects the character of each malt whisky. The first wash distillations produce a low level of alcohol, which is then re-distilled in the spirit still. During this second distillation, the spirit, containing about 65% alcohol by volume, is collected in the spirit receiver. All the products of the distillation are passed through the spirit safe, to enable the still man to check the strength and quality of the spirit.

5.   *Maturation*: this is the ageing process. For maturation or ageing, the newly distilled, colourless spirit is kept in oak casks. Most of the character and flavour of whisky are formed during this process. By law, the minimum requirement is three years for whisky to mature, but most single malt whiskies are kept in wood (oak) for eight years or more. The type of warehouse, temperature management etc. also influence the flavour and the strength.

6.   *Packaging and distribution*: mature whisky is always bottled in glass bottles. Most distilleries nowadays use automated machinery with which large quantities of whisky are bottled. A moving conveyer belt is used, on which the glass bottles are cleaned, filled, capped, sealed, labelled and lastly placed in cardboard boxes. Finally, the bottles are shipped and despatched.

WHAT ARE THE HEALTH ISSUES?

There are risks of physical injuries while manually handling, lifting or carrying, or from slipping, tripping, falling from a height or being hit by moving machinery, flying or falling objects. Heavy manual-handling-related musculo-skeletal disorders, work-related upper limb disorders (WRULD) and noise-induced hearing losses are some of the known occupational health risks. Harmful effects are also associated with exposure to hot liquids, cleaning substances etc. Alcohol vapour is highly inflammable, creating a fire hazard. Occupational lung disorders from exposure to grain and malt dust can occur. Coopering is the trade of making whisky casks from long curved pieces of wood. Coopers' work-related health problems may include asthma, nasal cancer or upper limb disorders.

Chapter 20: Wine making

Wine is made from grapes and the most common botanical varieties are *Vitis labrusca* and *Vitis vinifera*. Wine is an alcoholic drink which is produced by the fermentation of the grapes. The frosty-looking skin of the grape (the bloom) attracts airborne yeast and enzymes that ferment the juice of the grape into wine. Wine grapes are generally green, pale yellow or ruby red, and when wine is made, the usual percentage alcohol content is 10–14% and the colour may be red, white or rosé (pink). Four categories of wine are available: *table wine*, *sparkling wine*, *fortified wine* and *aromatic wine*. The quality of wine usually depends on the quality of the grapes, how they are cared for, how they are picked and lastly how they are fermented. Wines are also made from rice, palms, berries, cherries, apples, elderberries etc.; by the process of fermentation.

The history of wine making goes back to about 5000 BC in Egypt, as shown by the wine jars and paintings found in Egyptian tombs. The ancient Greeks and Romans also produced wines, and the Bordeaux region of France has been producing one of the best wines of the world for more than 2000 years. Gradually wine production started in Germany and other European countries instead of in Mediterranean countries only. The art of wine making reached the New World from Europe in the mid-1600s. From the nineteenth century onwards many states from America started to produce wine, and now California has become one of the largest wine producers in the world.

The process of wine making can be described in five stages:
1.   *Harvesting*: Wine grapes are harvested in autumn. Whether the grapes are ready for picking is usually determined by vineyardists, who inspect wine grapes using a refractometer. A refractometer is an instrument that determines the amount of sugar in the grapes. Once the grapes are ready, the picking is done by hand or by mechanical harvesters, robots etc. The mechanical harvesters gather and funnel the grapes into a field hopper or mobile storage container. The field hoppers or storage containers are then transported to the winery.

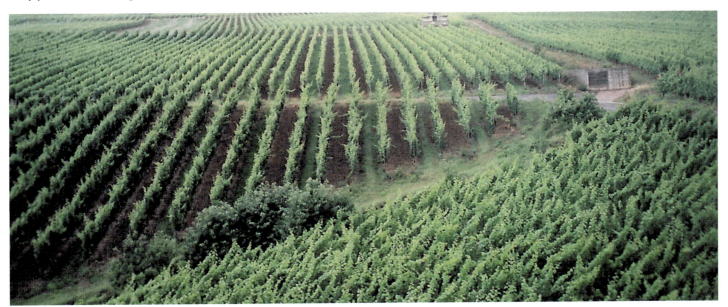

Vineyard in Rhine valley (Germany)

2.   *Grape crushing*: In the winery the grapes are unloaded from the field hoppers or mobile storage containers into a crushing machine. The grapes are crushed and the stems are removed. The crushed grapes are called must.

3.   *Fermentation*: The next step is fermenting the must. For white wine, all the grape skins are separated from the must by filtration or centrifugation prior to fermentation.

For red wine, the whole crushed grape, including the skin, goes into the fermentation tank or vat. During the fermentation process, wild yeast is fed into the tank or vat to turn the sugar in the 'must' into alcohol. Cane or beet sugar may be added to increase the alcohol content. Sugar content in the tank or vat is usually measured by a hydrometer. To increase the strength, various degrees of yeasts may be added. The fermentation process usually takes 1–2 weeks, depending on the type of wine being produced.

4.   *Storing, racking, filtering and aging the wine*: After fermentation, wine needs to be stored in a cool place. Large wineries now store wine above ground in epoxy-lined stainless steel tanks, though many wineries still store it in damp, subterranean wine cellars. The tanks are temperature-controlled by water, instead of the old redwood or concrete vats where wine is temporally stored during the settling process. The settling process is called racking and the wine is then pumped into racking tanks or vats for 1–2 months. Racking is done at 6–10°C (50–60°F) for red wine and 0°C (32°F) for white wine. After the initial settling (racking) process, certain wines are pumped into another settling tank or vat where they are kept for another 2–3 months. During settling the weighty, unwanted debris settles at the bottom of the tank and the wine is pumped into another tank. After the settling process the wine passes through a number of filters or centrifuges: the object of the filtering process is to remove unwanted sediments. After filtering the wine is aged in stainless steel tanks or wooden vats or barrels. Red wine is kept for 7–10 years, white and rosé for 1–4 years. Wine is either kept in large, temperature-controlled stainless steel tanks above ground, or stored in wooden barrels in damp wine cellars.

5.   *Bottling and packaging*: After aging, the wine is bottled, corked, sealed, labelled, crated and distributed. Wine bottles have corks made from special oak. The corks are covered with peel-off aluminium foil or plastic seal. Some wine bottles have an aluminium screw cap or plastic stopper. Some wineries use automated bottling machines. Finally, wine is usually shipped in wooden crates or packaged in cardboard.

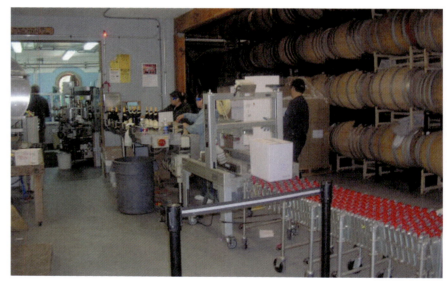

Winery in California's Napa Valley, USA

WHAT ARE THE HEALTH ISSUES?

Wines makers and winegrowers can develop respiratory-related rhinitis and asthma. Besides asthma, winegrowers can develop alveolitis, acute bronchial irritation syndromes and fibrosis and these can all be classified under 'winegrower's lung'. Cases of pesticide-related respiratory disorders have also been reported. Carbon dioxide poisoning can occur from inhaling toxic carbon dioxide during the fermenting process. Fermentation of grapes releases carbon dioxide, which is heavier than air and therefore sinks to the ground. It is important to keep any wine-making facilities well ventilated. Physical injuries from noise, tools, harvesting, and machinery, including cuts, falls etc., can occur. Recently, three wine makers were found dead inside a 1.5-metre (5-foot) deep wine tank in Coimbra, Portugal.

BOOK 1: ALREADY PUBLISHED AND AVAILABLE NOW

It contains the following 20 chapters:

1. Bangles
2. Basket making
3. Brass and metal working
4. Brick making
5. Carpet making
6. Coffee
7. Embroidery
8. Glass making
9. Lace making
10. Lavender
11. Leather
12. Mask making
13. Paper making
14. Plastics
15. Pottery making
16. Rope making (non-metallic)
17. Rubber
18. Sewing
19. Sugar cane
20. Tea

BOOK 3: COMING SOON

It contains the following 20 Chapters:

1. Beadwork
2. Beer making
3. Block printing
4. Boat building
5. Candle making
6. Cheese making craft
7. Fireworks
8. Fishing industry
9. Flowers
10. Hydrofoils and Hovercraft
11. Kite making
12. Lock making
13. Paintings
14. Pedicure and Manicure
15. Pearls and Amber
16. Potpourri
17. Scaffolding
18. Sculpture
19. Sholapith craft
20. Totora Reeds work

Lightning Source UK Ltd.
Milton Keynes UK
UKIC01n1043260414
230636UK00009B/39